# DRUGS & BEYOND

## A Family Approach To Abused & Misused Drugs

### By Global Health Research

## "Drugs and Beyond"

## This publication contains reference information only It is in no way intended to be prescriptive or diagnostic.

This book is a reference work based on extensive research. The intent is to offer wiser choices, natural alternatives, and solutions for the multitudes addicted due to the abuse and misuse of prescription or illegal drugs. In the event you use this information without your doctor's approval, you are prescribing for yourself, which is your constitutional right, but the publisher and author assume no responsibility.

1st Edition - Copyright © 1994 Global Health Ltd.
2nd Edition - Copyright © 1995 Global Health Ltd.

Global Health Ltd.
Box 18, Site 1, RR2
Tofield, Alberta, Canada
T0B 4J0

Canadian Cataloging in Publication Data
Drugs & Beyond
Includes Bibliographical References and Index
1. Drugs -- Physiological effect. 2. Drug abuse -- treatment.
I Global Health Research Foundation. II Global Health Ltd.
HV5801.D78 1994   362.29   C94-910599-6

ISBN 0-921202-10-5

Printed in United States of America

# How To Use This Book

This book will provide you, the reader, with valuable information on drugs, used for medicinal purposes or otherwise, which have the potential for dependency, abuse and/or misuse. It is set up in an easy to use format to avoid the frustrations commonly caused by disorganized manuals.

This section will give you general information on how to use this book to its fullest capacity. Immediately following this passage is a list showing the format, and a description of each specific category.

**Name:** in this category, you will find the name of a specific drug and information on what it is.

**Derivatives:** this category will list the chemical name(s) of each specific drug or drugs.

**Brand Names:** this category will not only list the chemical name, but by what name it is known to the consumer.

**Street Names:** this category consists of a list of common street names used by abusers to avoid speculation of abuse.

**Medical Advantages:** in this category is a list of how these drugs are used in medicine.

**Illegal Applications:** in this category, you will find a brief description on the use of a drug or drugs of any form that, if caught doing so, he/she will be treated as a criminal and will be prosecuted accordingly.

**Appearance and Methods Of Use:** this category will tell you what the drug(s) look like and how they are used.

**Behavioral Characteristics:** in this category is a list of characteristics which an abuser may have so that others can recognize the person as an abuser and provide any necessary help or actions which will aid in the victims withdrawal and recovery.

**Short Term Effects:** this is a list of symptoms which may be set on by the drug(s), but only last until the drug's(s') effects have worn off.

**Long Term Effects:** this category will list irreversible effects caused by the misuse of a drug or drugs.

**Tolerance and Dependence:** in this category, one will find whether tolerance is built through the use of the drug(s), whether psychological and/or physical dependence is developed and symptoms of withdrawal which are set on by the drug(s) with a dependency potential.

**Helpful Natural Treatments:** this category will list how a person using a drug(s) can heal him or herself with the use of supplements, foods and herbs.

# DEDICATION

The staff at Global Health dedicate this work to all people struggling with the problem of drug abuse and those who have encountered a previous loss of a family member or loved one due to the misuse of drugs. We also extend gratitude to the many foundations, support organizations, and their dedicated employees who have worked so hard to inform the general population on the misuse of drugs and the problems they cause.

# ACKNOWLEGEMENTS

Global Health expresses sincere appreciation to Shane Weatherill, of Edmonton, Alberta for the excellent artwork, cover design, and the illustrations interspersed throughout this manual. Particular gratitude is extended to Mark Rosin, Wayne Chemney and David Nyholt for the library research, typeset, and text design. We also wish to thank the Global Health research staff for their time, energy and support in the preparation of this book.

# FOREWORD

This is an informative, heavily researched book which has been construed by some of the top drug specialists. The purpose of this book is to help you fully understand about drugs, their uses and how they affect you and your children.

Drugs play a large part in our present day world. There are over-the-counter drugs that will fight off pains, strains and aches. Drugs which will help a person sleep and drugs that will keep a person awake. The list of drugs is never ending, as new drugs keep being discovered and each of them having their own qualities and uses; medicinal or otherwise.

Some drugs have properties that will make people feel and do things they normally wouldn't. For example, certain drugs may change moods, personalities, common human functions, etc. Drugs of this type are quite often abused or misused and are commonly referred to as illegal, illicit, abused or misused drugs or substances.

People often use these drugs as a sort of "escape route" from their problems in the "real world". When people have trouble dealing with reality or when life becomes too difficult, they turn to an artificial means of dealing with their problems. The downfall to these drugs is, in most cases, they are very addictive and, when abused, these drugs can hurt the body physically and can make a person mentally unstable due to the need for the drug(s).

This book will explain the uses, good and bad, and the short and long-term effects these drugs have on people. It will also explain how addictive the different drugs are, how they are used (medically and illegally), and give you a general idea about what each drug is. Furthermore, if someone is addicted to a drug, this book will show this person how he/she can help themselves get off of the drug(s) and onto a better lifestyle and physical self.

# *"Drugs and Beyond"*

## QUICK REFERENCE INDEX

# WHAT IS...?

**A DRUG** - is any foreign substance that alters the function of one or more body organs or changes the process of a disease. Drugs include prescribed medicines, over-the-counter remedies, and substances, such as alcohol, tobacco, and drugs of abuse, that are not used for medicinal purposes.

**DRUG ABUSE** - is taking a drug or drugs for purposes other than which the drug or drugs were intended, and/or the illicit use of a drug or drugs which can cause harm (not necessarily physical) to oneself and/or to others.

**DRUG MISUSE** - is the use of a drug for a purpose other than that for which it is normally prescribed or recommended. Among the many reasons for drug misuse are the desire to escape from reality, to achieve a mystical experience, curiosity about a drugs effects, the search for self-awareness and/or a better understanding of life and its meaning.

**DRUG ADDICTION and DEPENDENCE** - is the compulsion to continue taking a drug, either to produce the desired effects that result from taking it, or to prevent the ill effects that occur when it is not taken (withdrawal symptoms).

**DRUG TOLERANCE** - is the body adapting to the presence of a drug. When the tolerance to a drug increases, more of the drug is necessary to achieve the same effect.

**AN ILLEGAL APPLICATION OF DRUGS** - is the use of a drug or drugs of any form that, if caught doing so, the accused will be treated as a criminal and will be prosecuted accordingly.

# DRUGS AND YOUR FAMILY

The best time to prevent drug abuse is before it begins. However, the potential for drug experimentation and abuse among children is always present and should not be taken lightly. Each parent must learn to talk and develop good listening skills with their child or children. Sometimes it is not what is being said, but what is *not* being said. Unhappiness, loneliness and anxiety are often felt by a drug user, although he or she will not talk to his or her parents about the problems. Although many of them would like to have their parents' understanding, they feel they cannot approach their parents with such problems; usually out of fear of having to admit there is a problem and not knowing their parent's(s') reactions.

Pay attention to what information (even if it does not seem important at the time) your child or children give you. Does your child have new friends? Do you really know who they are? A parents close attention and a good relationship to your child or children is very important throughout the teenage years.

How can you tell, for sure, that your child is using drugs? Other than physical evidence, such as a high, there are signs that may indicate abuse. Keep in mind, though, that the following are not definite signs but only a sort of guide to tell that something is troubling your child.

Many children grow up hating school and will think of excuses to stay home or just not go to school. Check with school authorities and your child's teachers: do the days they missed because of being sick or otherwise, match what days you know they have missed?

What about missed classes? Being late for or skipping school or classes could be another tell-tale sign of a problem.

An extreme drop in grades can be a concern for a parent along with an "I don't care" attitude.

Other things to look for are temper tantrums, the child is very moody and gets angry over little things, and the child being disrespectful and not listening to authority figures in or out of school. A child's physical health can also play a part in discovering if your child is abusing drugs. When children are young, they usually have a lot of energy. If the energy seems to start disappearing and they are sleeping more and for longer hours (especially on weekends or holidays), coupled with a constant cough could be another sign of abuse.

Appearance is of utmost importance to a young adult. Children like to follow fads and other clothing or appearance trends. If your child's appearance is of little importance to him or her, pay attention and maybe approach them on it.

Children enjoy their privacy and will go to great lengths to protect it. However, if your child goes to extremes as not to let you in their rooms or doesn't let you know where he or she is going with his or her friends, this is a good sign your child is a drug abuser. Also, unexplained and lengthy stays of privacy in the bathroom cannot be ignored, especially if other behavioral changes are observed.

If your child asks you for money without an explanation for the use of the money, it may be to buy drugs.

Extreme character changes in your child could also be of significance. For example, if your child enjoyed, and was really good at a certain sport or sports and suddenly up and quit for no apparent reason.

Adolescents need to feel secure about communicating with their parent/s in which they feel they can approach them on anything without feeling threatened or blamed. As children get older, they find it difficult to share personal feelings with their parents and prefer to share their feeling with friends or other people in their age group. Although many parents know this, you should still try to have them be able to trust and confide in you. Constant and open communication is the key to a child's trust.

Understanding and forgiveness is what most children want in the relationship with their parents. Even if they know they are in trouble of some sort, they want to know that they can approach their parent(s) or guardian(s) and get the help and understanding they need and have come to you for.

# ABUSED DRUGS

| Drugs | Is/Are... | Tolerance Developed |
|-------|-----------|---------------------|
| **Amphet-amines** | Artificial stimulants related to adrenalin, a natural substance in the body, which speed up the processes of the body. | Some tolerance to amphetamines is possible and one should be cautious when using these drugs for medical purposes or otherwise. |
| **Alcohol (ethyl alcohol or ethanol)** | A colorless liquid known as ethanol or ethyl alcohol which is the active ingredient in alcoholic beverages such as beer, wine and hard liquors (spirits). | Tolerance is possible, especially in the chronic user. This may lead to addiction and, therefore, should be treated with caution. |
| **Anabolic Steroids** | A group of synthetic hormones similar to the natural male hormone testosterone. Steroids are most often used by athletes wanting to improve their performance, especially in sports requiring strength and power. | None. |

| Physical and Psychological Dependence | Physical and Psychological Long Term Effects | Impaired Judgments |
|---|---|---|
| Little physical dependence is developed, but psychological dependence is prevalent and should be treated with caution. | Long term effects are very probable with extended use, the worst having to do with the mind, i.e.- chronic psychosis and repeated talking. | Judgments are impaired and should not be taken lightly. Higher doses create higher impairment and should be avoided if mental awareness is a must, i.e.- driving, operating heavy machinery, etc. |
| Psychological and physical dependence are developed rather quickly and severely in the chronic user and should not be taken lightly. | There are effects, both psychological and physical. Many of them are irreversible and should be treated with caution. | Judgments are definitely impaired and, in fact, most countries have banned the consumption of alcohol while or before driving or operating of heavy machinery. |
| Psychological dependency occurs because the drug user uses it daily and it becomes habitual. They usually feel that without the drug, they will never be able to keep the body tone and size they now have. This is not true. All it takes is a lot more time and dedication, but the end result can be the same. | Include: aggressiveness, cardiovascular complications, liver disorders, heart disease and other complications, baldness, stunted growth, and male characteristics in females. | None. |

# ABUSED DRUGS *continued*

| Drugs | Is/Are... | Tolerance Developed |
|-------|-----------|---------------------|
| **Barbiturates** | A class of drugs which act as sedatives or induce sleep. | Yes. Especially when taken in repeated short intervals. |
| **Benzodiaze-pines** | Drugs which bring tranquillity by calming, soothing, quieting, or pacifying without depression. | Yes, when taken in repeated short intervals. |
| **Cocaine and Crack** | Are stimulants. Cocaine can be used as a local anesthetic, where crack (a smokable form of cocaine) is used only for abuse. | Tolerance can be developed over time. |

| Physical and Psychological Dependence | Physical and Psychological Long Term Effects | Impaired Judgments |
|---|---|---|
| Physical dependence develops with extended use of around 1 to 2 months or more. Psychological dependence also exists because of the minimal side effects. | Shortened memory, constant drowsiness, loss of coordination and awareness, emotional instability, slurred speech, and paranoia. | Yes. |
| Physical dependence can be developed over time and psychological dependence may be developed because of the minimal side effects. | Shortened memory, constant drowsiness, loss of coordination and awareness, emotional instability, slurred speech, and paranoia. | Judgments are impaired due to the sleep inducing effects. |
| Physical dependence may also be developed, especially if the user is injecting or smoking the drug. Psychological dependence may also be developed. It may be achieved when the user uses it as a way to deal with stress. | Regular use may cause: restlessness, anxiety, suspiciousness, insomnia, severe cardiovascular complications, hallucinations, and delusions, weight loss, constipation, impotence, difficulty in urination, and possibly lethargy and apathy. | Judgments can be impaired, especially in high dosages. |

# ABUSED DRUGS continued

| Drugs | Is/Are... | Tolerance Developed |
|---|---|---|
| **DMT (dimethyl-triptamine)** and **DET (diethyl-triptamine)** | Are both chemical analogues of tryptamine, a substance found to exist in natural resources around the world.<br><br>DMT is an active ingredient in various South American snuffs and is found in nature, where DET has not.<br><br>It is not absorbed through the skin or bloodstream when in direct contact. For this reason, it is smoked or inhaled. | It is not known if tolerance to these tryptamine analogues is developed, but if it is, it is gradual due to its short duration of effects which can last from about 20 minutes to around 1 hour. |
| **Inhalants** | Substances such as glue, nail polish remover, and gasoline which can be sniffed to produce mind-altering effects. | Yes, and as they sniff more of the drug, they produce the same harmful effects, but on a larger scale. |
| **LSD** | A derivative of an acid extracted from ergot, a rye grain fungus called Claviceps purpurea. LSD is colorless, tasteless, and odorless with a potency being compared to one ounce having the ability to be divided into 300, 000 doses. | Yes. As doses are increased, there are no differences on a person's mind or feelings, but the damaging effects on the body still continue. |

| **Physical and Psychological Dependence** | **Physical and Psychological Long Term Effects** | **Impaired Judgments** |
|---|---|---|
| There is no physical dependence developed, but some psychological dependence is possible. | Include: cardiovascular complications due to inhalation of the snuff or s moke.<br><br>Other problems may be developed if it is taken by injection. | Hallucinations and confusional syndrome may impair judgments. |
| There is little physical dependence, but a higher chance of psychological dependence. | Memory loss, brain damage, personality changes, tremors, nerve damage, muscular weakness, fatigue, nausea, vomiting, and problems associated with the liver, kidneys, eyes, bone marrow, heart, and blood. | Yes. |
| In some people, some psychological dependence may be developed. | Depression, anxiety, and flashbacks. There are, however, possibilities of suicides, accidental deaths, birth defects, miscarriages, murders, and self-inflicted wounds. | Yes. |

# ABUSED DRUGS continued

| Drugs | Is/Are... | Tolerance Developed |
|---|---|---|
| **Magic Mushrooms** | Of the family of fungi. Muscimole, psylocibyn and psilocin are thought to be the active principles responsible for the effects caused by the different types of mushrooms. | Tolerance can be developed by these mushrooms to the point where they have no effect. |
| **Marijuana and Its Derivatives** | A mood-altering drug from the leaves of the cannabis sativa plant which possesses hallucinogenic effects. | None. |
| **Morning Glory & Wild Woodrose Seeds** | Used as intoxicants and as hallucinogens. | Tolerance is developed quite quickly. |

| Physical and Psychological Dependence | Physical and Psychological Long Term Effects | Impaired Judgments |
|---|---|---|
| There is no physical dependence developed to this type of drug. There may be minor psychological dependence, but this will usually occur in only a choice few. | Cardiovascular problems may develop if it is smoked. | Yes. Distortion of size, color and sound all add to misjudgments. |
| There is little, if any physical dependence developed, it is almost all due to psychological dependence. | If it is being smoked, chances of contracting lung diseases, such as cancer, are increased. Also, lack of personal hygiene, slow mental responses, and lessened communication skills. | Judgments are slowed. |
| There is no physical dependence developed, but psychological dependence is possible. | Depression, anxiety, and flashbacks. There are, however, possibilities of suicides, accidental deaths, birth defects, miscarriages, murders, and self-inflicted wounds. | Judgments are definitely impaired and if under the influence, operation of heavy machinery and / or driving should be avoided. |

# ABUSED DRUGS *continued*

| Drugs | Is/Are... | Tolerance Developed |
|---|---|---|
| **Opiates** | Painkilling drugs which may produce a sense of well-being and euphoria; they are also referred to as narcotic analgesics or opiate narcotics. | None. |
| **PCP (Phencyclidine or Sernyl)** | An anesthetic and hallucinogen. | Tolerance is developed from the use of phencyclidine. |

| Physical and Psychological Dependence | Physical and Psychological Long Term Effects | Impaired Judgments |
|---|---|---|
| All the opiates and opiate substitutes have potential for dependence. The craving or compulsion to take the drug is strong, especially with the purest forms such as morphine, heroin and china white. | Decreased sexual drive, constipation, and menstrual irregularity. If one is injecting, chances of infections, liver disease, ulcers, phlebitis, extensive scarring, AIDS, and other complications, are increased. Also, birth complications such as breech delivery, higher rates of miscarriage, premature birth, and the possibility of the baby being born addicted are not uncommon. | None. |
| Physical and psychological dependence is not uncommon in the chronic user. | Because of its anesthetic properties, bodily harm can occur without the user realizing it before it is too late. Persistent speech problems, depression, anxiety, birth complications, memory loss, flashbacks, aggressiveness, violence, paranoia, delusions, and auditory hallucinations may also occur. | Yes. |

# ABUSED DRUGS continued

| Drugs | Is/Are... | Tolerance Developed |
|---|---|---|
| **Peyote (Mescaline)** | Peyote is a gray-green spineless cactus with a dome-shaped head having tufts of whitish hair and a long, carrotlike root. Mescaline is the drug responsible for most of peyote's effects. | None. |
| **Phenothia-zines** | The most widely used drugs for problems associated with psychoses. | No tolerance has been noted. |
| **PIA's** | Amphetamine analogues of mescaline which produce effects of both hallucinogens (at high doses) and amphetamines (at low doses). | Tolerance is developed quite quickly to the phenyisopropylamines. |

| Physical and Psychological Dependence | Physical and Psychological Long-Term Effects | Impaired Judgments |
|---|---|---|
| None. | A possibility of psychological damage with extended use. | Yes. |
| None. | If severely abused, these drugs can cause the following: bone and brain damage and severe kidney, lung, liver, heart, and muscle disorders. | Because of the immediate effects caused by these drugs, judgments may be impaired. |
| These drugs do not produce physical dependence, but psychological dependence may be mildly developed, especially if taken in low doses for its amphetaminelike effects. | Brain damage from overdose and severe convulsions is possible, as is death, although these are not common. | Judgments are definitely impaired which makes operation of any vehicle, or any other task for that matter, a challenge and increase the risk of harm to oneself and to others. |

# ABUSED DRUGS *continued*

| Drugs | Is/Are... | Tolerance Developed |
|---|---|---|
| **Quaaludes (Methaqualone)** | Non-barbiturate sedative-hypnotics. They act on a different central nervous system sites than other sleeping pills, such as barbiturates. | Yes. Tolerance is developed quickly to use in the day and at night. |
| **Tobacco (Nicotine)** | Is an annual plant of the nightshade family. It is a stimulant, in small doses, but depresses in larger doses. | Tolerance is developed over time. |

| Physical and Psychological Dependence | Physical and Psychological Long Term Effects | Impaired Judgments |
|---|---|---|
| Physical and psychological dependence are both developed through the use of methaqualone. Although physical dependence is strong, psychological dependence is even stronger. | Brain damage, cardiovascular complications, and coma from overdose which could lead to death. | Yes. |
| Physical dependence is developed over time and although, in a cigarette, it is mild, it becomes habitual which makes the user even more dependent on this drug. | Cancers, heart disease, and damage to the cardiovascular system. | None. |

## "Drugs and Beyond"

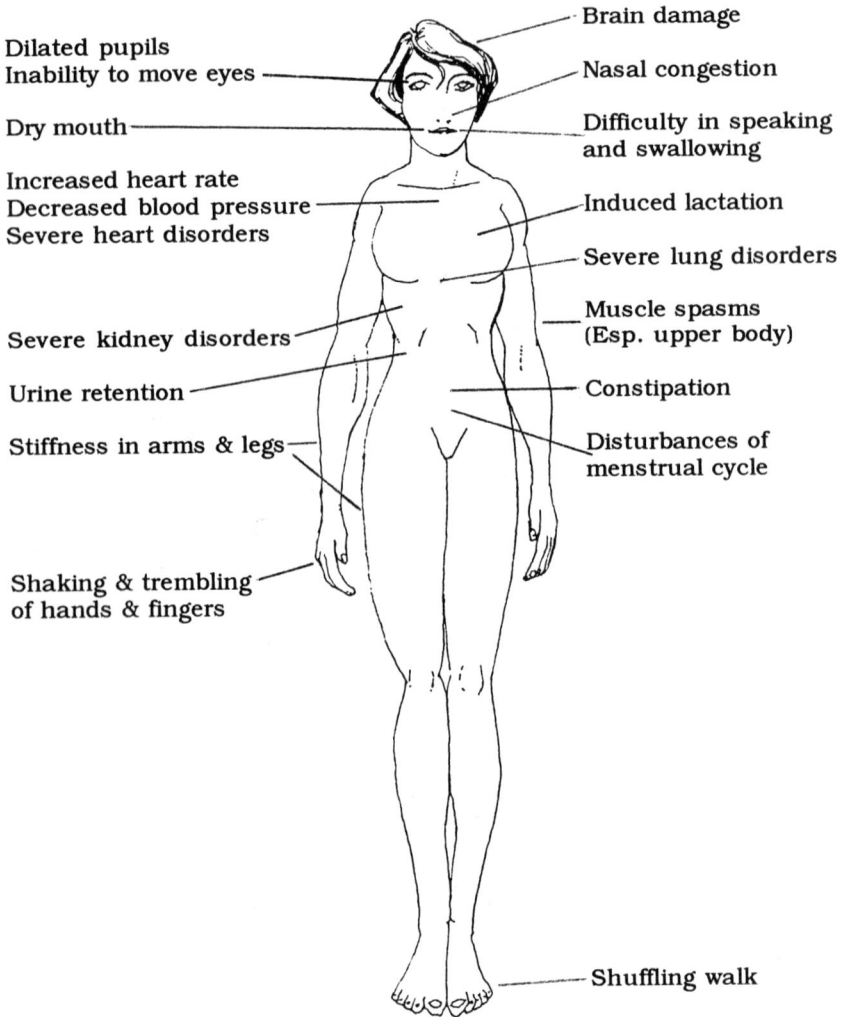

Brain damage

Dilated pupils
Inability to move eyes

Nasal congestion

Dry mouth

Difficulty in speaking
and swallowing

Increased heart rate
Decreased blood pressure
Severe heart disorders

Induced lactation

Severe lung disorders

Severe kidney disorders

Muscle spasms
(Esp. upper body)

Urine retention

Constipation

Stiffness in arms & legs

Disturbances of
menstrual cycle

Shaking & trembling
of hands & fingers

Shuffling walk

Adverse effects and problem areas associated
with short and long term use of
**Antipsychotic Agents (tranquilizers)**

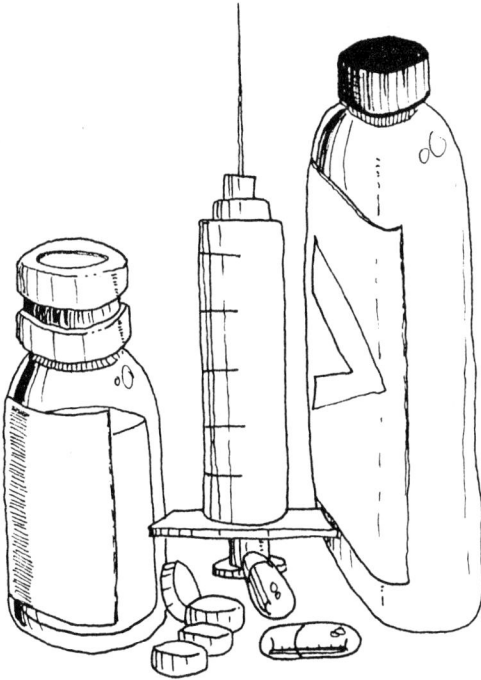

## *ANTIPSYCHOTIC TRANQUILIZERS*

**Phenothiazines** - are the most widely used drugs for the problems associated with psychoses. They are used to treat emotional, mental, metabolic and nervous disorders and to treat such ailments as anxiety, agitation, pain, severe hiccups, severe nausea and vomiting and severe itching.

**Haloperidol (Haldol)** - is not a phenothiazine, but has similar properties. A major difference is that it is metabolized and excreted at a much faster rate. Haloperidol can be used as an alternative for patients who may be unresponsive to phenothiazines and for symptoms of Tourette's disorder.

**Derivatives:** *phenothiazines:* acetophenazine, chlorpromazine, fluphenazine, mesoridazine, methotrimeprazine, pericyazine, perphenazine, pipotiazine, prochlorperazine, promazine, thiopropazate, thioproperazine, thioridazine, trifluoperazine, triflupromazine. *Haloperidol.*

# "Drugs and Beyond"

**Brand Names:** *Acetophenazine:* Tindal; *Chlorpromazine:* Chlorpromanyl-5, Chlorpromanyl-20, Chlorpromanyl-40, Largactil, Largactil Liquid, Largactil Oil Drops, Novo-Chlorpromazine, Ormazine, Thorazine, Thorazine Concentrate, Thorazine Spansule, Thor-Prom; *Fluphenazine:* Apo-Fluphenazine, Modecate, Modecate Concentrate, Moditen Enanthate, Moditen HCl, Moditen HCl-H.P., Permitil, Permitil Concentrate, Prolixin, Prolixin Concentrate, Prolixin Decanoate, Prolixin Enanthate; *Mesoridazine:* Serentil, Serentil Concentrate; *Methotrim-eprazine:* Levoprome, Nozinan, Nozinan Liquid, Nozinan Oral Drops; *Pericyazine:* Neuleptil; *Perphenazine:* Apo-Perphenazine, PMS Perphenazine, Trilafon, Trilafon Concentrate; *Pipotiazine:* Piportil L4; *Prochlorperazine:* Compa-Z, Compazine, Compazine Spansule, Cotranzine, PMS Prochlorperazine, Prorazin, Stemetil, Stemetil Liquid, Ultrazine-10; *Promazine:* Primazine, Prozine-50, Sparine; *Thiopropazate:* Dartal; *Thioproperazine:* Majeptil; *Thoridazine:* Apo-Thioridazine, Mellaril, Mellaril Concentrate, Mellaril-S, Novo-Ridazine, PMS Thioridazine; *Trifluoperazine:* Apo-Trifluoperazine, Novo-Flurazine, PMS Trifluoperazine, Solazine, Stelazine, Stelazine Concentrate, Terfluzine, Terfluzine Concentrate; *Trifluprom-azine:* Vesprin.
*Haloperidol:* Apo-Haloperidol, Halodol, Halodol Decanoate, Halodol LA, Novo-Peridol, Peridol, PMS Haloperidol.

**Street Names:** Unknown, but most likely called by name.

**Medical Advantages:** these drugs are used for the treatment of psychoses. The absence of Dopamine in the brain, results in Parkinson's disease, but when levodopa, in possible combination with carbidopa, is used it replaces the Dopamine, thus, accepted treatments for this disease. In schizophrenic patients, phenothiazines can reduce hostility, paranoia, suspiciousness, uncooperativeness, and social incompetence.

**Illegal Applications:** purchasing, consuming, prescribing or selling these drugs without authorization from proper authorities.

**Appearance And Methods Of Use:** orally as tablets, oral concentrate, syrup, elixir, oral solution, oral suspension, or as extended - release or other capsules. Also by injection or as suppositories.

**Behavioral Characteristics:** agitation, dizziness, drowsiness, change in color vision, congested nasal passages, blurred vision, long periods of time spent in the washroom due to constipation, tremors, difficulty in speaking or swallowing, inability to move eyes, masklike face, muscle spasms, shaking or trembling of the hands, staggered and shuffling walk. Also see "Short Term and Long Term Effects" for further evidence of abuse.

**Short Term Effects:** dry mouth, dilated pupils, drowsiness, nasal congestion, blurred vision, constipation, retention of urine, tremors, may cause the body to produce less sweat creating a feeling of extreme warmth which may cause discomfort, increased heart rate, change in color vision, difficulty in speaking or swallowing, difficulty in seeing at night, inability to move eyes, masklike face, loss of balance control, restlessness or a need to keep moving, stiffness in arms or legs, twisting movements of the body, muscle spasms (especially the upper body), shuffling walk, ticlike or twitching movements, shaking or trembling of the hands and fingers, dilation of blood vessels resulting in decreased blood pressure, especially if the person rises from a reclining position.

They may also affect certain hormones; they may disturb the menstrual cycle, and may induce lactation (secretion of milk from the breasts) in women who are not pregnant which may lead to swelling or pain in the breasts.

Rare side effects are convulsions, fast heartbeat or irregular pulse, high or low blood pressure, loss of bladder control, unusually pale skin, difficult or fast breathing, fever, increased sweating, severe muscle stiffness and unusual tiredness or weakness.

**Long Term Effects:** severe kidney, heart, liver, muscle, lung disorders, coma and possibly death; possible bone weakness and brain damage if severely abused.

**Tolerance and Dependence:** tolerance, physical dependence and psychological dependence are not developed.

### Helpful Natural Treatments:

*Vitamins:* A, B, B2, B3, B5, B6, B9, B12, B complex, C, Sodium ascorbate (buffered vitamin C), and E.

*Minerals:* Calcium, Magnesium (chelate form), Selenium and Potassium.

*Aminos:* L-Glutathione, L-Lithium carbonate & L-Phenylalanine.

*Herbs:* Astragalus, Cowslip, Echinacea, Ginseng, Licorice Root, Lobelia, Milk Thistle, Siberian Ginseng, Golden Seal, Suma, Valerian Root, and Red Spearmint is used to safely alleviate restlessness associated with withdrawal symptoms.

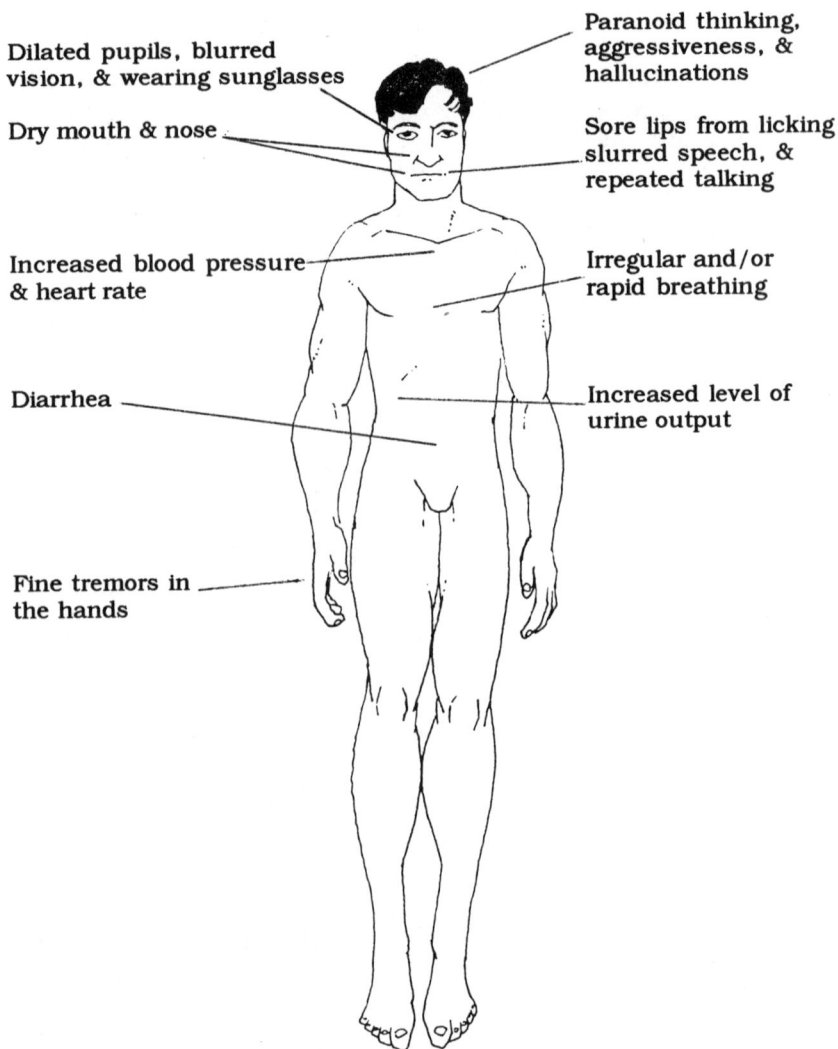

Dilated pupils, blurred vision, & wearing sunglasses

Paranoid thinking, aggressiveness, & hallucinations

Dry mouth & nose

Sore lips from licking slurred speech, & repeated talking

Increased blood pressure & heart rate

Irregular and/or rapid breathing

Diarrhea

Increased level of urine output

Fine tremors in the hands

Adverse effects and problem areas associated with short and long term use of **Amphetamines (behavioral stimulants)**

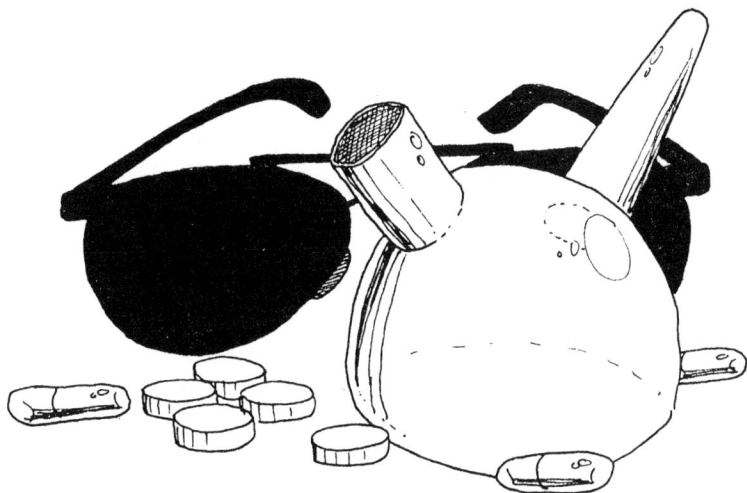

## BEHAVIORAL STIMULANTS
## and CONVULSANTS

**AMPHETAMINES** - are synthetic stimulants which are related to adrenalin. Adrenalin is a natural substance in the body which alerts the body; speeds up the processes of the body.

The action on the neurotransmitter system in the brain is thought to be the cause of the mood-altering effects of amphetamines. They cause increased release of dopamine and norepinephrine from brain cells, and block both their uptake and the activity of the enzyme responsible for metabolizing them. The increased levels of those neurotransmitters are the cause of many of the behavioral effects peculiar to this type of drug.

**Derivatives:** Amphetamine (also Amfetamine), Amphetamine and Dextroamphetamine Resin Complex, Dextroamphetamine (also Dexamfetamine), Methamphetamine (also Methamfetamine).

**Brand Names: Amphetamine:** Amphetamine; **Amphetamine and Dextroamphetamine Resin Complex:** Biphetamine, Biphetamine 121/2, Biphetamine 20; **Dextroamphetamine:** Dexedrine, Dexedrine Spansule, Oxydess II, Spancap; **Methamphetamine:** Desoxyn, Desoxyn Gradumet.

# "Drugs and Beyond"

Amphetaminelike drugs' brand names are: **Methylphenidate:** Ritalin, Ritalin-SR, Ritalin SR.

Appetite suppressants' brand names are: **Benzphetamine:** Didrex; **Diethylpropion:** M-Orexic, Nobesine-75, Tenuate, Tenuate Dospan, Tepanil, Tepanil Ten-Tab; **Mazindol:** Mazanor, Sanorex; **Phendimetrazine:** Adipost, Anorex, Appecon, Bacarate, Bontril PDM, Bontril Slow-Release, Dital, Dyrexan-OD, Marlibar A, Melfiat-105 Unicelles, Metra, Neocurb, Obalan, Obe-Del, Obeval, Obezine, Panrexin M, Panrexin MTP, Parzine, Phendiet, Phendiet-105, Phendimet, Phentra, Plegine, Prelu-2, PT 105, Rexigen, Rexigen Forte, Slyn-LL, Statobex, Tega-Nil, Trimcaps, Trimstat, Trimtabs, Wehless, Wehless-105 Timecells, Weightrol, Wescoid, X-Trozine, X-Trozine LA; **Phentermine:** Adipex-P, Dapex-37.5, Fastin, Ionamin, Obe-Mar, Obe-Nix, Obephen, Obermine, Obestin-30, Oby-Trim, Panshape, Phentercot, Phentride, Phentride Caplets, Phentrol, Phentrol 2, Phentrol 4, Phentrol 5, T-Diet, Teramin, Wilpowr, Zantryl.

Appetite suppressants are sometimes abused or misused because, first of all, they help, in this case young adults, keep a slim and trim body. Adolescents sometimes feel that if they are not trim and slim, they are not beautiful or handsome, and they will be stereotyped or misconceived as an outcast and nobody will like them.

They are also abused or misused because they have amphetaminelike properties. This will keep the person awake and, if they are attending school, may be used as a means of being able to learn better.

The problems associated with these uses are that a tolerance is built to their stimulant properties and the user become physically and psychologically dependent on them. This is a bad combination because as more is needed to produce the same effects, the more dependent one becomes. This may lead to the need for a stronger drug, like amphetamines, and soon their life will revolve around the need for the drug. This is of course not prevalent, but one should be aware of their abuse potential.

**Street Names:** Bennies, crank, black beauties, blackbirds, blue angels, caplets, chris/christine, crisscross, crossroads, crystal, dexies, double-cross, footballs, greenies, hearts, ice, kitty kat, LA ice, lidpoppers, ludies, mets, meth, mini beenies, mollies, peaches, pep pills, pinks, pocket rockets, rosas, sky rockets, sparkle, speed, splash, plenties, thrusters, truck drivers, uppers, ups, wake ups, water, whites.

**Medical Advantages:** doctors use amphetamines to treat conditions such as narcolepsy (uncontrolled sleeping episodes), a form of epilepsy called petit mal epilepsy, severe depression unresponsive to antidepressant drugs, pain relief (in conjunction with narcotic drugs), motion sickness, parkinsonism unresponsive to other drugs and urinary incontinence.

Amphetaminelike drugs, such as Ritalin (methylphenidate) and Cylert (pemoline) are used to treat hyperactive children or ADHD (attention-deficit hyperactivity disorder). Amphetamines increase attention and decrease restlessness in children who are overactive, unable to concentrate for very long or are easily distracted, and have unstable emotions. These drugs improve behavioral and learning ability in 50 to 75 percent of children correctly diagnosed of having such disorders. However, the use of behavioral stimulants is discouraged for "problem children" since many clinicians feel that large numbers of children diagnosed as having such disorders are incorrect.

In addition, it is common that the family situation of these children has frequently occurring episodes of depression in one or more parents. It is hypothesized that the children exhibit these behaviors as a natural defense mechanism against his or her own state of depression.

Amphetamines were used as "diet pills", but a tolerance to the appetite-suppressant action appears within about 2 weeks, thus, the dose must be increased to continue the effectiveness of the amphetamine drug. Once tolerance is developed, and unless the dose is increased to the point of the user becoming agitated, the person usually resumes his or her previous eating pattern and gains back all the lost weight. As a result, amphetamines are no longer recognized as effective drugs for long term control of obesity.

**Illegal Applications:** smokable methamphetamine crystals (Ice, LA Ice, Crank) is a fairly new drug which, when produced, has a high profit margin. In the United States, one pound of Ice (which costs around $700 to produce) has a street yield of $225 000. Obviously, this is why it is more attractive to the drug dealer. And to the user, it is attractive for its long lasting effect which surpasses Crack's by 14 hours or more.

Also, the selling, consuming, purchasing or prescribing amphetamines without authorization from proper authorities.

**Appearance And Methods Of Use:** taken orally. Methamphetamine crystals are smoked.

# "Drugs and Beyond"

**Behavioral Characteristics:** sore lips from constant licking when the user is high, drop in grades, constant cough, increased illness, change of friends, unusual borrowing of money, loss of interest in former goals, sloppy dress, wearing sunglasses because of the annoying brightness of light and irritability to motion due to dilated pupils, mood swings, weight loss, loss of personal possessions (sold to buy drugs), difficulty in concentrating and slurred speech.

Also see "Short Term and Long Term Effects" for further evidence of abuse.

**Short Term Effects:** Increased alertness, insomnia, shakiness, rise in blood sugar level, increased blood flow to musculature, decreased blood flow to internal organs, increased blood pressure and level of urine put out, breathing can become rapid or irregular, the mouth and nose can become dry, diarrhea, loss of appetite, constant licking of the lips, dilated pupils, a need for sweet and cold products, a lack of personal cleanliness, blurred vision, high fever and muscle spasms. Depression, irritability, panic, paranoid thinking, confusion, hallucinations, aggressiveness, convulsions, high fever, psychotic behavior, incoherent speech and coma may occur in high dosage use and can last up to 48 hours.

A rise in blood pressure, increase in pulse rate, dilated pupils (and the gaze may be fixed, glossy or normal), anorexia, increased blood glucose and coagulability, increased skeletal muscle tension, dry mouth and difficulty swallowing solid food, cool skin from narrowing of blood vessels closest to the outer skin, increased deep tendon reflexes, fine tremors in the hands, urinary retention and constipation may also occur.

Increased doses may cause anxiety, speech is rapid, slurred and incoherent. motions may be fidgety, jerky and random.

Teeth grinding is possible as are thoughts being loosely connected.

**Long Term Effects:** Chronic sleep disorders, irregular heartbeat, high blood pressure, skin rash, suppressed appetite, nutritional and speech problems and repeated talking. Chronic psychosis, a condition similar to paranoid schizophrenia, is possible of occurring when amphetamines are used for a prolonged period of time.

*Tolerance and Dependence:* some tolerance is developed through the use of amphetamines. Dependence is developed to the drug after chronic use, even in low doses. After stopping use of the drug, extreme fatigue sets in. The sleep that follows is usually disturbed, but gets better after a few days. A large appetite and moderate to severe depression are typical of withdrawal from amphetamines. Kainic acid may play a role in the future of amphetamine withdrawal treatment since, depending on the amount given, it can increase or decrease the effects amphetamine has on the body.

Symptoms of overdose are a high fever, extreme dizziness, difficulty breathing, increased blood pressure, convulsions, coma and possibly death if not treated immediately.

### Helpful Natural Treatments:

*Vitamins:* A, B3, B5, B12, B complex, C, Sodium ascorbate (buffered vitamin C) and E.

*Minerals:* Calcium, magnesium (chelated form) and Selenium.

*Aminos:* L-Glutathione, L-Lithium carbonate & L-Phenylalanine
Foods: dark green leaves, flax, hemp seed, pumpkin seed, soy bean and walnut.

*Herbs:* Astragalus, Cayenne, Cowslip, Echinacea, Ginseng, Hops, Licorice Root, Lobelia, Milk Thistle, Pau D'Arco, Siberian Ginseng, Golden Seal, Suma, Valerian Root, and Yucca.

*Also:* a high potency miltivitamin; a high potency mineral complex; a Protein supplement; GABA (gamma-aminobutyric acid); Linolenic acid; Red Spearmint. This herb can be used to safely alleviate restlessness associated with withdrawal symptoms.

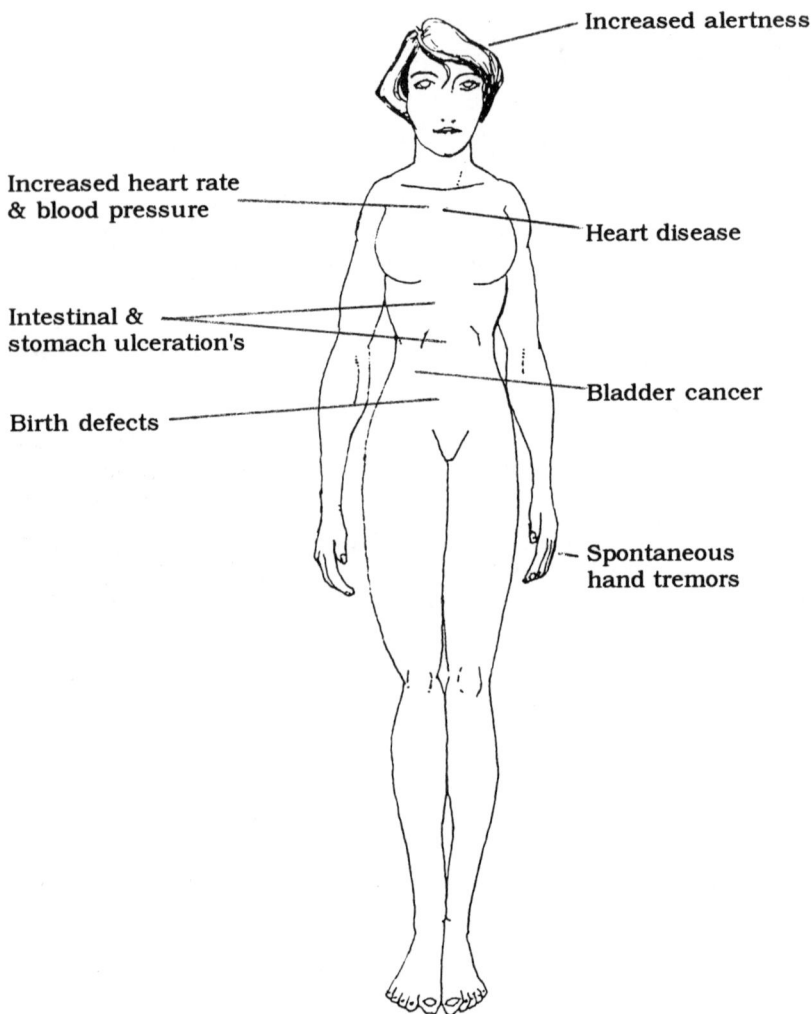

Increased alertness

Increased heart rate
& blood pressure

Heart disease

Intestinal &
stomach ulceration's

Bladder cancer

Birth defects

Spontaneous
hand tremors

Adverse effects and problem areas associated
with short and long term use of
**Caffeine**

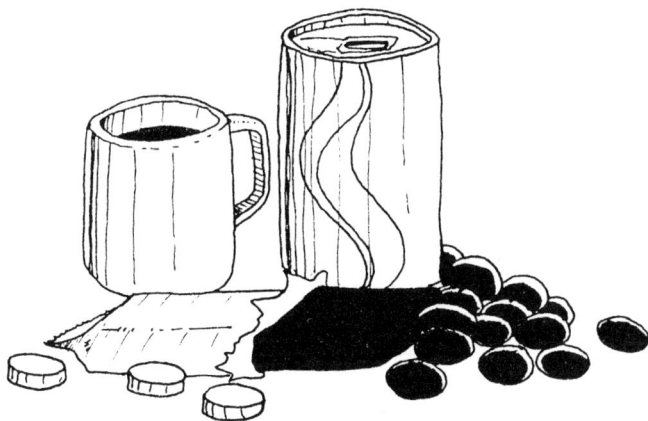

## CAFFEINE

**CAFFEINE** - is a stimulant and a diuretic (helps form and expel urine from the body) which, in coffee, comes from the coffee bean or the Coffea arabica plant; though there are many other sources of caffeine. The average 5 oz. cup of coffee contains between 80 to 120 mg. of caffeine, although instant coffee contains from 70 to 100 mg. Thus, different processes and brands of coffee contain different strengths of caffeine.

**Derivatives:** coffee, tea, cocoa, cola drinks, compound headache preparations, cold preparations, "stay-awake" pills.

**Brand Name:** all commercial trade names.

**Street Names:** brew, coffee, pop, soda, soda pop, tea.

**Medical Advantages:** since caffeine constricts cerebral blood vessels in humans, it is good for headaches if the cause of them is due to expansion of blood vessels in the brain.

**Illegal Applications:** none.

**Appearance And Methods Of Use:** drank as a beverage, taken in a tablet form or eaten (as in chocolate or otherwise).

**Behavioral Characteristics:** mood swings caused by the lack of sleep due to the overconsumption of caffeine. Also see "Short Term and Long Term Effects" for further evidence of abuse.

# "Drugs and Beyond"

**Short Term Effects:** increased alertness, heart rate and systolic and diastolic blood pressures; insomnia; irregular heart beat in some individuals; spontaneous tremor of hands.

Caffeinated coffee also increases alertness during the day, but it is also proven that, when drunk at night, it has a considerable effect on alertness.

**Long Term Effects:** if a person drinks 8 or more cups of coffee a day, it can cause effects such as insomnia, anxiety, stomach and duodenal ulceration, heart disease, bladder cancer and a possibility of birth defects.

**Tolerance and Dependence:** tolerance is not developed through the use of caffeine, but dependence is possible, especially when it is used to "wake up" in the morning. Withdrawal from caffeine can cause irritability, restlessness, headache.

Symptoms of overdose or caffeine poisoning are extreme agitation, an abnormal cardiac rhythm, seizures and possibly even death. These symptoms can appear after 25 to 50 cups of coffee, although the amount considered toxic varies from individual to individual.

### Helpful Natural Treatments:

*Vitamins:* A, B complex, B1, B2, B3, B5, B6, B9, B12, C, Sodium ascorbate (buffered vitamin C) D, E and K.

*Minerals:* Calcium, Iron, Magnesium (chelated form), Potassium, Selenium and Zinc.

*Aminos:* L-Glutathione, L-Lithium carbonate & L-Phenylalanine.

*Herbs:* Astragalus, Cayenne, Cowslip, Echinacea, Ginseng, Hops, Licorice Root, Lobelia, Milk Thistle, Pau D'Arco, Siberian Ginseng, Golden Seal, Suma, Valerian Root, and Yucca.

*Also:* a high potency multivitamin; a high potency mineral complex; a Protein supplement; Red Spearmint. This herb can be used to safely relieve restlessness associated with withdrawal symptoms.

Violent behavior

Dilated pupils

Chapped nostrils &
hole in barrier

A stuffy, sore
or bleeding nose

Rapid respiration

Chest pain &
lung damage

Rapid heart rate

Track marks

Tremors & twitching

Impotence &
difficult urination

Constipation

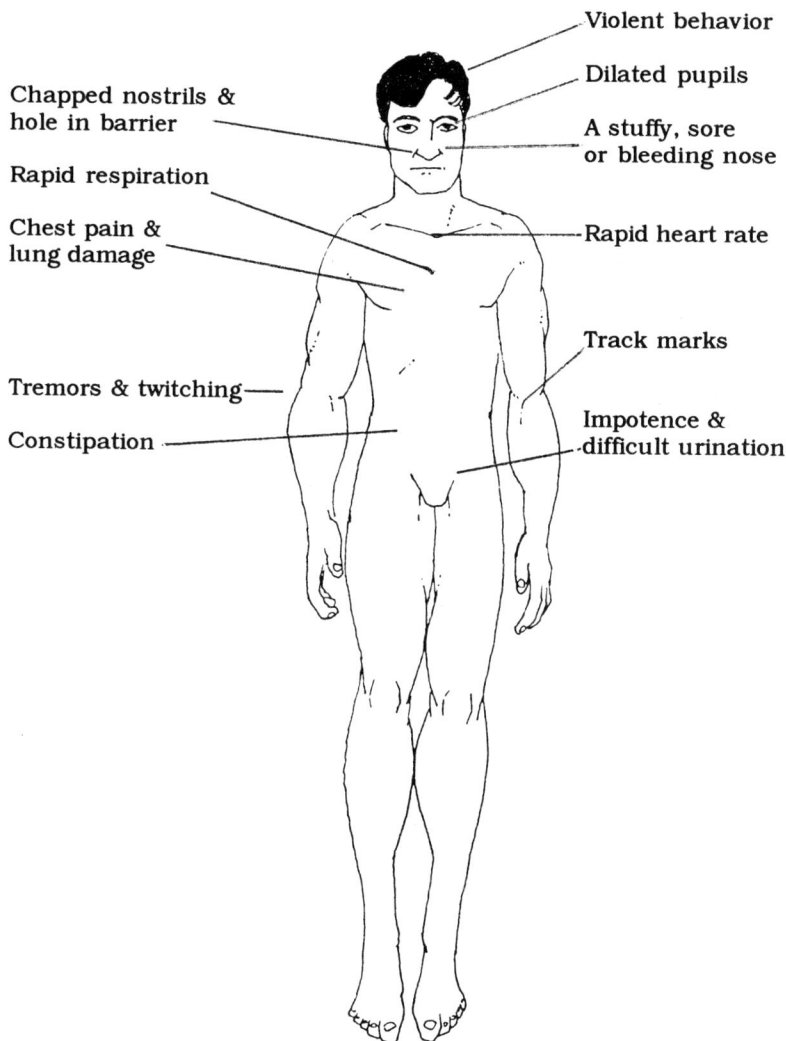

Adverse effects and problem areas associated
with short and long term use of
**Cocaine/Crack**

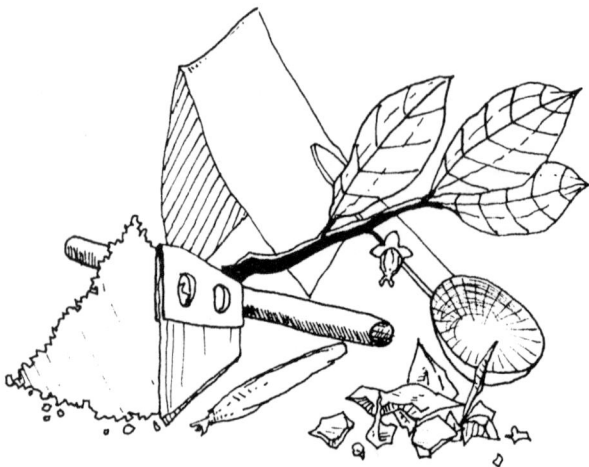

## COCAINE

**COCAINE (benzoylmethylecgonine)** - is a local anesthetic - a drug that, when applied to mucous membranes or injected about nerves, produces a loss of sensation, a stimulant - a drug that speeds up the central nervous system and a narcotic.

It is obtained from the leaves of the Erythroxylum coca shrub. Usually sold as a fine white powder, the drug is sometimes cut or diluted with substances which look similar to it, such as icing sugar or cornstarch. Also, it is sometimes mixed with products, such as lidocaine or benzocaine, which mimic the numbing effects of cocaine. This means that the buyers of the drug are not always getting what they pay for.

Coca paste is the first product in the production of cocaine. Although not very pure, coca paste can contain from 40 to 85 percent cocaine along with a number of other solvents used in the extraction process. The behavioral effects coca paste can produce are identical to that of cocaine's.

Crack is a form of cocaine which can be smoked. It is called "crack" because of the cracking sound it makes during both processing and smoking. It is made with pure cocaine and common household products which are dissolved, shaken with water and the remaining solid substance is crack. People find smoking crack provides a better, more intense high than snorting or sniffing cocaine powder, but is also more susceptible to dependence and overdose.

Cocaine was once considered the drug which identified the rich from the poor; or the drug of the elite. The reason was the high cost for a "high". This is no longer true. Even though the cost of cocaine is still very pricey, there is no specific group of people who have surrendered to the addicting effects of cocaine.

**Derivatives:** cocaine hydrochloride.

**Brand Name:** mucosal-local.

**Street Names:** *Cocaine* - blanco, blow, C, caine, coca, coke, cola, croke, dream dust, flake or flakes, girl, girl toot, gold, gold dust, heaven dust, lady, Lady Line Muser, nose candy, paradise, perico, Peruvian Flake, polvo, she, snow, stardust, toot, white, white lady, white girl.
*Crack* - bazooka, crack, crystal, french fries, fry daddle, moonrock, ready rock, rock, space base, space cadet, tar, tragic magic.

**Medical Advantages:** cocaine is used as a local anesthetic.

**Illegal Applications:** the manufacturing, selling, purchasing and/or using cocaine/crack/coca paste/coca leaves without authorization from a proper authority.

**Appearance And Methods Of Use:** methods of use are snorting through the nostrils, injecting, free basing (smoking), and/or chewing or swallowing the leaves of the coca plant. A typical dosage does not really exist since the user will usually spend all the money he/she has on hand, on cocaine and continue administering it until it is gone. Smoking and injecting cocaine produce more intense effects than snorting. In order for the typical street cocaine to be smoked, it must first be treated chemically.
Coca paste (an impure substance which contains 40 to 85 percent cocaine and other products from the extraction process) is free based (smoked) as a cigarette.
Crack can be smoked in a pipe; crushed, mixed with tobacco and smoked as a cigarette or can be mixed with water and injected. Inhaling the smoke introduces the cocaine directly into the lungs and subsequently into the left side of the heart, bypassing the veins. It takes 6 to 8 seconds to cause an effect. Lasting only minutes, the high is intense. As a comparison, when snorting cocaine the effect does not peak until 15 to 40 minutes after the dose.

# "Drugs and Beyond"

**Behavioral and Physical Characteristics:** irritability, aggressive behavior, delirium, hallucinations, psychosis (including paranoid behavior), unusual borrowing of money, loss of personal possessions (sold to buy drugs), drop in grades, sloppy dress, burn holes in clothes, mood swings, constant cough, increased illness, change of friends, wearing sunglasses or the use of visine (to hide the redness of the eyes), constant consumption of junk food and pop or other flavored beverages, weight loss, loss of interest in former goals, strangely long fingernails (usually the pinkie nail) used to scoop and snort the cocaine crystals, difficulty in concentrating, may have slurred speech, a desire to talk constantly and move about, if the user administers the drug by sniffing, the nostrils will constantly be running, or sometimes the user will have the illusion that his/her nose is running, and there will be an ulceration in the cartilage separating the nostrils. Also see "Short Term and Long Term Effects" for further evidence of abuse.

**Short Term Effects:** people under the influence of cocaine generally feel more confident, energetic and alert. Physical effects include a rapid heartbeat and respiration, increased body temperature, dilated pupils, sweating, mild hearing loss (not permanent), paleness and decreased appetite. Large quantities can cause unusual or violent behavior, tremors, loss of coordination, twitching, hallucinations, pain or pressure in the chest, nausea, blurred vision, fever, muscle spasms, convulsions, high blood pressure and stroke. Users of cocaine can get a "hangover" which may cause insomnia and a stuffy nose.

Most fatal overdoses result from respiratory failure due to seizures, heart failure or stroke. Death from cocaine is more likely to occur when the drug is smoked because of the extremely rapid rise in the level of cocaine in the blood.

**Long Term Effects:** regular cocaine users are often restless, extremely excitable, suspicious, and suffer from insomnia, hallucinations and delusions, weight loss, constipation, impotence and difficulty in urination.

Continual heavy use eventually leads to lethargy, apathy and sleeplessness. Regular users often abuse other drugs to relieve these symptoms.

Characteristic signs of chronic cocaine sniffing are: nasal stuffiness, runny, sore or bleeding nose and chapped nostrils.

Damage to the lining of the nose is not uncommon and may include the development of a hole in the barrier separating the nostrils.

Severe cardiovascular complications are also very probable with extended use. Crack smokers may also suffer damage to their lungs from the cocaine vapors.

There is also a chance of contracting the AIDS virus through the sharing of syringes. To make matters worse, the use of cocaine can affect the outside of single nucleus blood cells in a way that it will increase HIV - 1 replication; in other words, the disease will spread more rapidly through the body.

Medical complications involve almost every organ system and curing cocaine addiction is difficult tedious work and should be done under specialized conditions.

**Tolerance and Dependence:** tolerance to cocaine can be developed over time. Regular users are at risk to becoming addicted. Users can develop a strong craving for the drug, especially if they have been injecting or smoking it.

There are two main reasons why crack users are at the risk of becoming addicted. First, the user experiences an intense and rapid high. The user will feel the effects of crack in less than ten seconds. Second, the equally intense feelings of depression, anxiety and irritability which follow the euphoric state. This depressed state is experienced within five to ten minutes of smoking crack. Both the initial rush or euphoria and the subsequent feelings of depression motivate the person to use the drug again.

A stimulation phase of increased alertness, feelings of sexual prowess, and euphoria are followed by a cocaine rush. The high is so pleasurable and perceptions are so distorted that the user quickly feels that anything can be accomplished. The user may use the pleasurable effects in order to cope with a stressful situation or situations. More frequent use may result for relief in such settings. When the drug is taken in other than social or recreational settings, the initial effects may give way to dysphoria, restlessness and irritability within 30 minutes. Depression often results from that state, which produces enough discomfort to necessitate a rapid return to the drug, hence, the user becomes an addict.

Withdrawal symptoms may include depression, fatigue, long, but restless sleep, irritability, violent tendencies, confusion, anger and a strong craving for cocaine.

Symptoms of overdose are increased heart rate and blood pressure, elevated body temperature, rupture of brain aneurysms, brain hemorrhage, seizures and convulsions, unconsciousness, coma, respiratory failure and death if not treated immediately.

# "Drugs and Beyond"

**Helpful Natural Treatments:**

*Vitamins:* A, B complex, B3, B5, B12, C, Sodium ascorbate (buffered vitamin C) and E.

*Minerals:* Calcium, Magnesium (chelated form) and Selenium.

*Aminos:* L-Glutamine, L-Glutathione, L-Lithium carbonate, L-Phenylalanine and L-Tyrosine taken along with the enzyme tyrosine hydroxylase.

*Herbs:* Astragalus, Cayenne, Cowslip, Echinacea, Ginseng, Hops, Licorice Root, Lobelia, Milk Thistle, Pau D'Arco, Siberian Ginseng, Golden Seal, Suma, Valerian Root, and Yucca.

*Also:* a high potency multivitamin; a high potency mineral complex; a Protein supplement; Red Spearmint. This herb can be used to safely relieve restlessness associated with withdrawal symptoms.

Destroys brain cells

Heart disease

Increased heart rate

Damaged lungs

Increased blood pressure

Increased respiration

Contraction of cancers throughout the body

Birth defects

Nicotine stained fingers

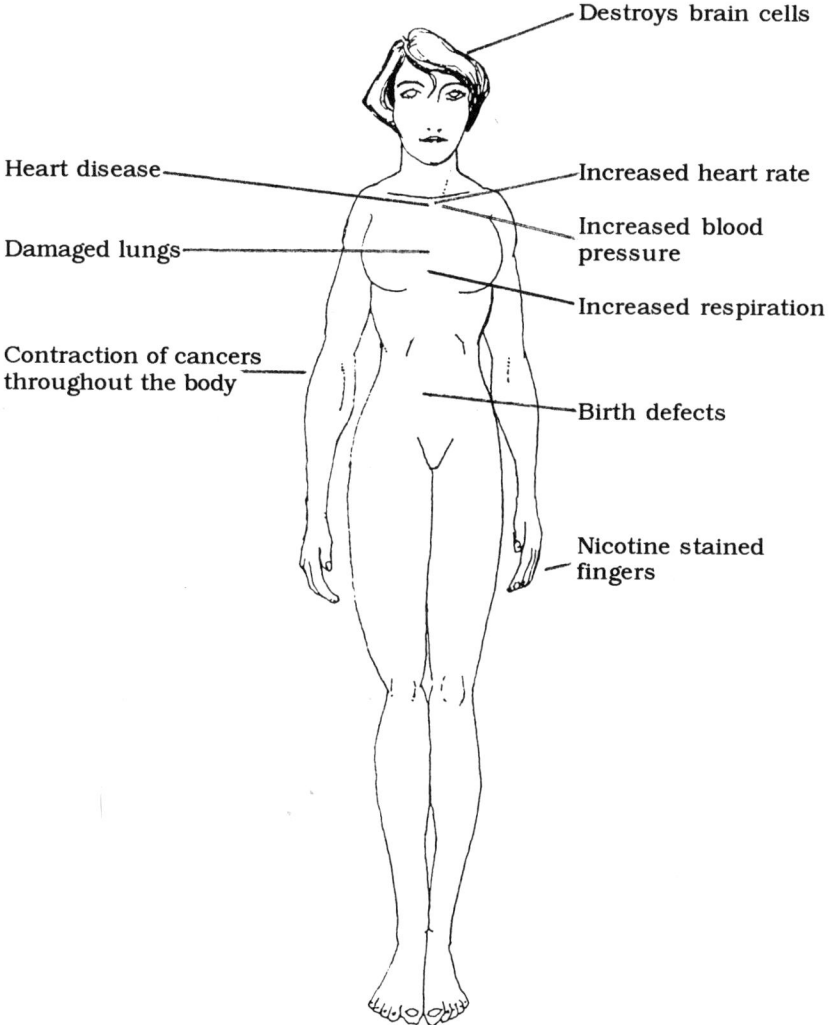

## Adverse effects and problem areas associated with short and long term use of
### *Tobacco*

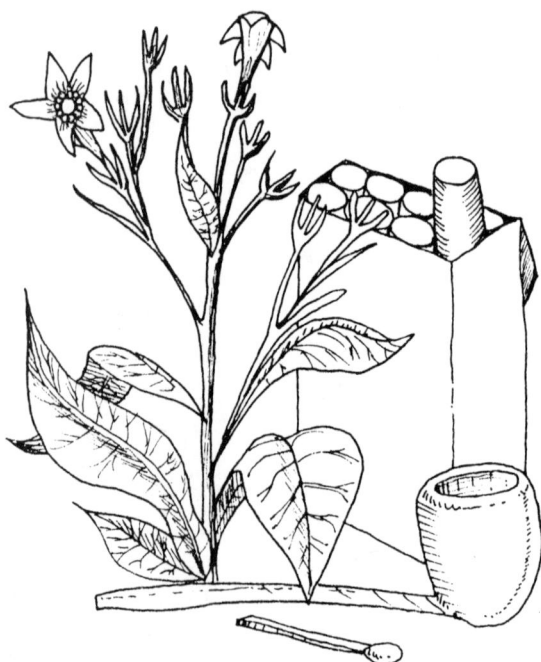

## *TOBACCO*

**TOBACCO** - is an annual plant from the nightshade family, whose leaves are prepared for smoking, sniffing and chewing. The alkaloid responsible for many of its effects is called nicotine. In small doses, nicotine first stimulates, but in large doses, depresses.

**Derivatives:** nicotine (C10 H14 N2); 1-Methyl-2-(3-pyridyl) pyrrolidine.

**Brand Name:** all commercial cigarettes, cigars, chewing tobacco, snuffs and manufactured processed tobacco. Prescription and nonprescription drugs with nicotine added; Habitrol, Nicoderm, Nicorette, Nicotrol, ProStep.

**Street Names:** snuff, smoke, gagger, spit, cancer sticks, stogie.

**Medical Advantages:** can be used to help fight asthma and keep the attacks to a minimum when used correctly.

Nicotine gum or "Nicorette" can be used to help discontinue the use of tobacco. Each piece contains 2 mg. of nicotine and should be chewed slowly for about 30 minutes. Generally, people find that 10 to 12 pieces are efficient per day.

**NOTE** - the gum should not be chewed if a person is pregnant or a nursing mother. It should definitely be kept out of reach of children.

The nicotine patch or "Habitrol (s(-)-Nicotine) is, yet, a further advancement in the area of nicotine addiction. Habitrol is designed to temporarily replace some of the nicotine that a cigarette would normally supply. It is available in 3 different strengths, 7 mg., 14 mg. and 21 mg. While the person wears the patch, controlled quantities of nicotine pass from the patch into your skin, and ending up in your bloodstream. Because some nicotine is left on the skin after the patch is removed, the nicotine will continue to enter the body for several hours afterwards.
Withdrawal from cigarette smoking is very real because of the bodies craving for nicotine. Studies have shown that nicotine provides a barrier that protects the brain from unpleasant or distracting external stimuli; in other words it acts as a sort of buffer for things like annoying noises, arguments or over stimulation of any kind. When a person quits smoking, the brain no longer has the nicotine buffer and withdrawal symptoms set in. These symptoms consist of frustration, dizziness, tiredness, craving for cigarettes, irritability, lack of concentration, sleep disturbances and increased appetite. It takes approximately 12 weeks for an ex-smoker to feel comfortable with the idea of living without the drug. For natural foods which help the body with withdrawal symptoms, see "Helpful Natural Treatments."

**Illegal Applications:** the selling of cigarettes to minors or the selling of contraband cigarettes.

**Appearance And Methods Of Use:** tobacco can be chewed, sniffed or smoked in a pipe or through a tube, but the most common way is to smoke it is as a manufactured cigarette or a hand rolled cigarette.

**Behavioral Characteristics:** unusual borrowing of money, burn holes in clothes, constant cough, increased illness, yellow or brown stains on fingers, cold room (frequent airing out) and a change of friends. Also see "Short Term and Long Term Effects" for further evidence of abuse.

# "Drugs and Beyond"

**Short Term Effects:** a person who smokes will have a constant cough as the lungs are trying to get rid of the unwanted phlegm, the heart will beat faster, blood pressure will increase and the level of carbon monoxide in the bloodstream will increase; binding to the hemoglobin, it will decrease the amount of oxygen in your system.

**Long Term Effects:** there is a risk of extremely increasing a persons chance of contracting cancers and heart diseases and permanently damaging the lungs and cardiovascular system. There is also a higher risk of birth defects.

Cigarette smoke contains about 4000 different chemicals including trace amounts of such poisons as DDT, arsenic and formaldehyde which can permanently harm the body.

**NOTE** - people who are constantly or even periodically around smokers are also at risk of contracting sicknesses and diseases. Second hand smoke has more carcinogenic tars than inhaled smoke. If you are one of these people, see "Helpful Natural Treatments" to help your body get rid of such poisonous toxins.

**Tolerance and Dependence:** a person's body will adjust to its own level of nicotine needed to function properly. Dependence develops rapidly and most addicts find they prefer to smoke more cigarettes of low nicotine levels rather than less of high nicotine level cigarettes.

Withdrawal symptoms include: anxiety, cravings for cigarettes, gastrointestinal complications, headaches, increased appetite, irritability, restlessness and sleeping disorders.

### Helpful Natural Treatments:

*Vitamins:* A, B, B complex, B3, B5, B12, C, Sodium ascorbate (buffered vitamin C), E.

*Minerals:* Calcium, Magnesium (chelated form) and Selenium.

*Aminos:* L-Glutathione, L-Lithium carbonate & L-Phenylalanine.

*Herbs:* Astragalus, Cayenne, Cowslip, Echinacea, Ginseng, Hops, Licorice Root, Lobelia, Milk Thistle, Pau D'Arco, Siberian Ginseng, Golden Seal, Suma, Valerian Root, and Yucca.

*Also:* Raw, unsalted shelled sunflower seeds which will decrease the acidity of the bloodstream in smokers, thus lessening the loss of nicotine. By chewing the seeds, a person will find that he or she will not have to light up or chew as often and it will supply the oral gratification by giving your mouth something to do.

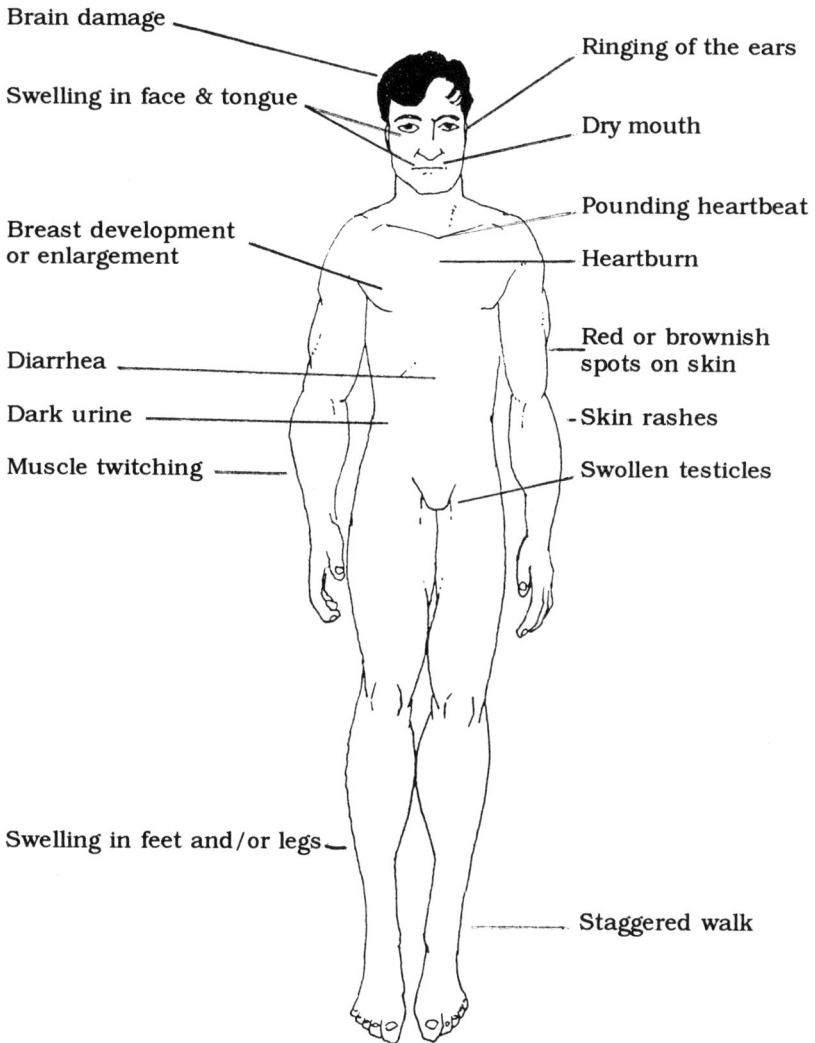

Brain damage

Swelling in face & tongue

Breast development
or enlargement

Diarrhea

Dark urine

Muscle twitching

Swelling in feet and/or legs

Ringing of the ears

Dry mouth

Pounding heartbeat

Heartburn

Red or brownish
spots on skin

Skin rashes

Swollen testicles

Staggered walk

Adverse effects and problem areas associated
with short and long term use of
*Clinical Antidepressants*

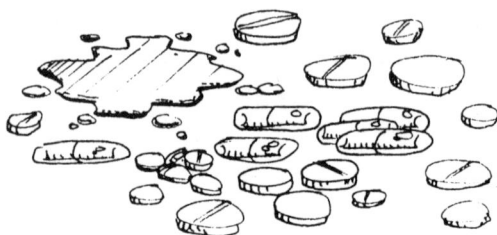

# CLINICAL ANTIDEPRESSANTS

These drugs are used for such mental disorders as depression and mania in which they help stabilize and elevate mood.

Depression is described as one who has feelings of hopelessness, sadness, and a general loss of interest in life accompanied by a sense of reduced emotional well-being. Depression is not caused by one single factor. It can be caused by one or more of many factors. These factors include hormonal disorders; lack of communication with a loved one (like a father-son relationship); physical illness; such outside disturbances as the loss of a job or loved one or a change in the weather or season; or even a drug which will depress the body or change regular hormonal production.

People who are depressed, will usually find that the symptoms gradually go away as the day goes on. In other, more severe cases, the symptoms seem to be worsened over night and the affected person will be withdrawn from the outside world and may spend their days huddled in bed.

Mania is a form or phase of mental disorder in which there are extreme feelings of joy or rage, uncontrolled and often violent activity, extravagant and irregular speech and is often followed by depression. It usually occurs as part of manic depression as well. In some cases, mania will accompany depression. This disorder is called manic-depression and a major contributing factor is that it can be inherited.

Manic depression is described as being a mental disorder in which there is a disturbance of mood. In some cases, severe mood swings (i.e. - irritability or anger) may be accompanied by extreme negative delusions, depression or sadness and far fetched ideas. There are two types of antidepressant drugs, tricyclic antidepressants and monoamine oxidase (MAO) inhibitors.

Tricyclic antidepressants are used to relieve mental depression. This type of antidepressant drug is abused, not usually by the patients, but more commonly by substance abusers. They use drugs like Amitriptyline (Elavil) and Doxepin (Sinequan) for their sedating properties which exist at high doses, but are more commonly used in combination with alcohol, benzodiazepines or narcotics which will enhance the sedating effects of these drugs.

MAO inhibitors are also taken to relieve certain types of depression and work by blocking the action of the enzyme known as monoamine oxidase in the nervous system.

Monoamine oxidase is a natural substance found in the body and plays an important role in regulating the central nervous system. It oxidizes and destroys neurotransmitters such as dopamine and other amines which have entered the body in drugs or any nutritionally valuable element in food, such as protein or carbohydrate.

Also, lithium can be used to treat people with manic-depressive illness. It is used to lessen the severity and number of manic states. Lithium is an alkali metal, like potassium and sodium. In the 1920' s, it was discovered to be a sedative-hypnotic compound, and 20 years later, was used as a salt substitute. Its use became disastrous as the consequences of its long term use were great, one consequence being death.

Today, technology and scientific research has given us a better understanding of drugs' effects and the capability to use drugs, like lithium, safely and properly.

Although research on these drugs is still being done to fully understand the reasons why antidepressant drugs are effective, it seems there is a functional deficiency of these amines in people with certain disorders. When MAO inhibitors are administered, they stop the action of MAO which results in giving the amines such as, serotonin, dopamine, and tyramine the capability to exist and do their job, thus, bringing the levels of these amines to the level at which they are most effective.

**Derivatives:** Monoamine Oxidase (MAO) Inhibitors: Isocarboxazid, Phenelzine, Tranylcypromine.

# "Drugs and Beyond"

Tricyclic Antidepressants are Amitriptyline, Amoxapine, Clomipramine, Desipramine, Doxepin, Imipramine, Nortriptyline, Protriptyline, Trimipramine.

In some cases, other drugs are occasionally classified and used as antidepressants since they possess properties and actions similar to those of the antidepressant drugs listed above.

**Brand Names: Isocarboxazid** - Marplan; **Phenelzine** - Nardil; **Tranylcypromine** - Parnate. **Amitriptyline** - Apo-Amitriptyline, Elavil, Emitrip, Endep, Enovil, Levate, Novotriptyn, PMS Amitriptyline; **Amoxapine** - Asendin; **Clomipramine** - Anafranil; **Desipramine** - Norpramin, Pertofrane; **Doxepin** - Novo-Doxepin, Sinequan, Triadapin; **Imipramine** - Apo-Imipramine, Impril, Janimine, Norfranil, Novopramine, PMS Imipramine, Tipramine, Tofranil, Tofranil-PM; **Nortriptyline** - Aventyl, Pamelor; **Protriptyline** - Triptil, Vivactil; **Trimipramine** - Apo-Trimip, Rhotrimine, Surmontil.

**Note:** *(For Monoamine Oxidase Inhibitors)* foods which have been aged, fermented or pickled, or which contain high concentrations of yeast, alcohol or caffeine may have severe adverse reactions and should be avoided when using these drugs.

The following applies to any of the drugs listed above:
any drugs, herbs or supplements being used (including other antidepressants) or ailments present prior to these medicines being prescribed should be told to your doctor to avoid any unnecessary adverse reactions.

**Street Names:** unknown.

**Medical Advantages:** given for relief of certain types of mental depression.

**Illegal Applications:** selling or consuming antidepressant and antimania drugs without permission from a proper authority figure.

**Appearance And Methods Of Use:** all are taken orally as capsules, oral solution, syrup or tablets with the exception of Amitriptyline and Imipramine which can also be taken by injection.

**Behavioral Characteristics:** mood swings, increased illness, change of friends, loss of personal possessions (sold to buy drugs), slurred speech, unusual eating habits especially of junk food and pop or other flavored beverages, drop in grades, unusual borrowing of money, loss of interest in former goals, staggered walk, and difficulty in concentrating. Also see "Short Term and Long Term Effects" for further evidence of abuse.

**Short Term Effects:** include: anxiety, dark urine, diarrhea, dry mouth, increased appetite, fever, nausea and vomiting, slurred speech, sore throat, staggered walk, irritability, being tired or weak, heartburn, weight gain, ringing of the ears, yellow skin or eyes, swollen testicles, convulsions, insomnia, poorly articulated speech, swelled feet or lower legs, swelling of face and tongue, quick or pounding heartbeat, muscle twitching, development of breasts in males and breast enlargement in females, mental confusion, lactation in females who are not pregnant, trouble with teeth and gums, red or brownish spots on the skin, skin rash and itching, severe dizziness, lightheadedness or head rushes, especially when sitting or standing up from a resting position.

**Note:** if any of the following are noticed, seek medical help immediately: increased sweating which may be caused by or lead to a fever, difficult or fast breathing, stiff or sore neck muscles, irregular blood pressure, pale skin, nausea and/or vomiting, convulsions, being unusually tired or weak, increased sensitivity to light, severe chest pain, loss of bladder control, slow or fast heartbeat, dilated pupils or severe headache.

**Long Term Effects:** are not common, but include cardiac failure and brain toxicity.

**Tolerance And Dependence:** tricyclic antidepressants produce mild physical dependence when these drugs are taken for prolonged periods of time. Tolerance to the anticholinergic effects is developed during prolonged treatment.

### Helpful Natural Treatments:

*Vitamins:* A, B, B complex, B3, B5, B12, C, Sodium ascorbate (buffered vitamin C) and E.

*Minerals:* Calcium, Magnesium (chelated form) and Selenium.

*Aminos:* L-Glutathione, L-Lithium carbonate & L-Phenylalanine.

*Herbs:* Astragalus, Cayenne, Cowslip, Echinacea, Ginseng, Hops, Licorice Root, Lobelia, Milk Thistle, Pau D'Arco, Siberian Ginseng, Golden Seal, Suma, Valerian Root, and Yucca.

*Also:* Red Spearmint can help to safely alleviate restlessness associated with withdrawal symptoms.

Slurred speech

Pinpointed pupils

Dry mouth

Impaired respiratory system

Moist, cold, & blue skin

Constipation

Liver disease

Track marks

Birth defects

Menstrual irregularity

Staggered walk

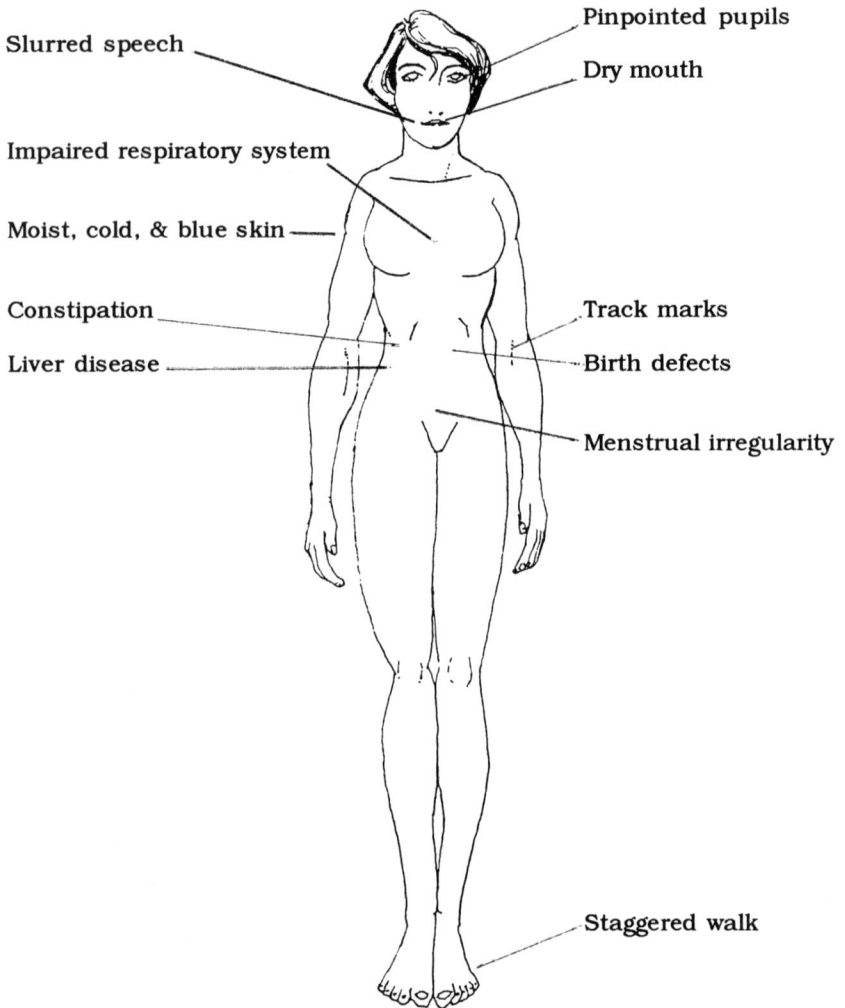

## Adverse effects and problem areas associated with short and long term use of
### *Opiate Narcotics*

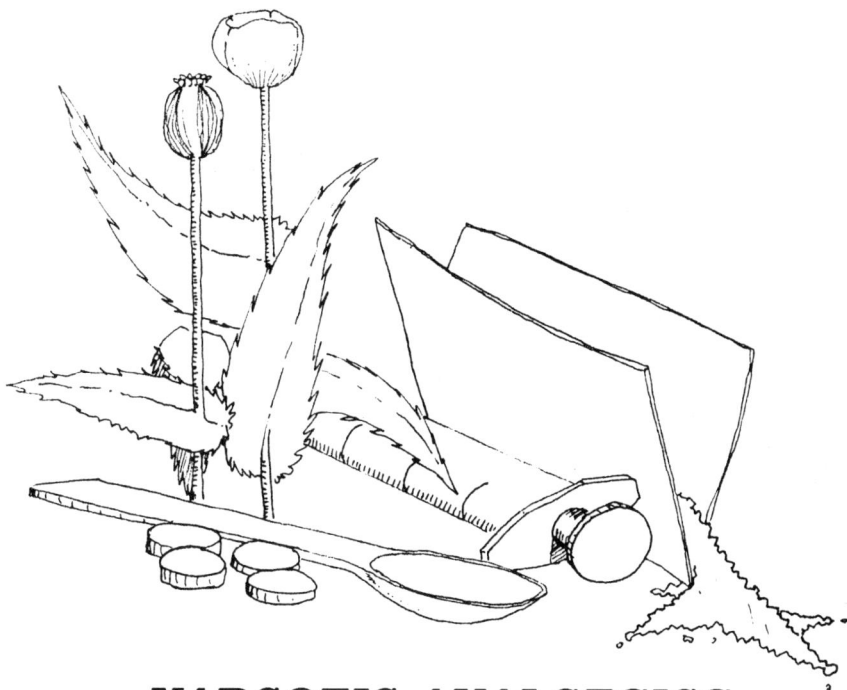

# NARCOTIC ANALGESICS
## (Opiates)

**NARCOTIC ANALGESICS** - are potentially addictive, kill pain and produce a sense of well-being and euphoria. Narcotic analgesics are also referred to as opiate narcotics, opiates and opioids.

Morphine and codeine are naturally occurring and are derived directly from the poppy plant (*Papaver somniferum*). Some, such as heroin, are chemically altered to produce stronger or milder effects depending on what its use is intended for. Others are synthetically produced and are not chemically related to the opiates. These have the same effects, but have different potencies and a much higher dependency potential.

Methadone, a synthetic drug, is used to treat heroin addiction and is about the same strength as morphine. Demerol (meperidine), also a synthetic narcotic, is only about 10 to 20 percent as potent as morphine.

# *"Drugs and Beyond"*

With one exception, all the compounds have a strong addiction potential. They all trigger analgesia and euphoria, and tolerance is built to them just as the other opiates. The exception is propoxyphene napsylate or Darvon. It isn't addicting, and won' t trigger analgesia or euphoria. At best, it is no more effective than aspirin, probably less so.

**Derivatives:** Morphine, Codeine.

**Brand Name: Alphaprodine** - Nisentil; **Anileridine** - Leritine; **Buprenorphine** - Buprenex; **Butorphanol** - Stadol; **Diacetylmorphine** - Heroin; **Diphenoxylate and Atropine** - Lomotil; **Fentanyl** - Fentanyl Citrate; **Hydrocodone** - Hycodan, Robidone; **Hydromorphone or Dihydromorphinone** - Dilaudid, Dilaudid-HP; **Levorphanol or Levorphan** - Levo-Dromoran; **Meperidine or Pethidine** - Demerol; **Methadone** - Dolophine, Methadose; **Methylmorphine** - Codeine, Paveral; **Morphine** - Astramorph, Astramorph PF, Duramorph, Epimorph, Morphine H.P., Morphitec, M.O.S., M.O.S.-S.R., M S Contin, MSIR, RMS Uniserts, Roxanol, Roxanol 100, Roxanol SR, Statex; **Nalbuphine** - Nubain; **Opium or Papaveretum** - Pantopon; **Oxycodone** - Roxicodone, Supeudol; **Oxymorphone** - Numorphone; **Pentazocine** - Talwin, Talwin-Nx; **Propoxyphene or Dextropropoxyphene** - Darvon, Darvon-N, Dolene, Doraphen, Doxaphene, Novopropoxyn, Profene, Pro Pox, Propoxycon.

**Street Names:**

**Diacetylmorphine** - big H, boy, brown, brown sugar, caballo, chinesett, chiva, crap, do-jee, dope, dragon, elephant, estuffa, gear, goods, H, hard stuff, Harry, heroina, hombre, horse, jive, junk, material, mexican mud, mud, No. 3, No. 4, nanoo, polvo, product, scag, scat, schmeck, smack, stofa, stuff, sugar, thing, tiger, white stuff.

**Fentanyl** - china white, down or downs, killer heroin, number four, powder, white poison, white powder.

**Hydromorphone** - first line.

**Morphine** - cube, hard stuff, morf, white stuff.

**Meperidine** - cube, demis, junk, white stuff.

**Methadone** - medicine dollies, biscuits.

**Opium** - op, poppy.

**Oxycodone** - morf, morfina, morpho, morphy, mud.

**Oxymorphone** - goma.

**OPIUM** - The sole source of opium is the head of the poppy, *Papaver somniferum*. Opium is "smoked" by being heated, not burned, and the smoke rising from it is inhaled. The usual practice is to take a small pellet of opium, heat it over a flame, place it in a pipe and inhale the smoke. Since opium doesn't vaporize very well, a specially prepared opium is always used.

Opium smoking is less likely to lead to dependency than the oral route (drank as a beverage; added to such liquids as laudanum or other liquid concoctions). Only about 10 percent of the morphine content is released in the vapor, and supposing that all this entered the bloodstream, a person would have to smoke about 8 grams of opium to get the equivalent of a typical one - third grain of a heroin street bag.

The more potent, or refined, the drugs are, the greater the problems. With opium it is not unusual for a person to keep the level stabilized for years. With morphine, such equilibrium is far more difficult to maintain, and heroin, even harder.

If we have learned anything from various societies, it is that people who use drugs in their natural forms have fewer problems than those who use refined drugs.

**CODEINE** - is one of two major alkaloids of opium, the other being morphine, used extensively in medicine. In equal doses it is 1/6 as potent as morphine. Doctors seem reluctant to prescribe the drug in pure form and prescribe drugs with codeine in them. These drugs are not as effective, more expensive and usually have unpleasant side effects, such as internal bleeding.

**FENTANYL (China White)** - is a synthetic opiate which, as a pain reliever, is about 80 times more potent than morphine and, as a street drug, is from 50 to 2 000 times more potent than street heroin. Alpha Methylfentanyl is an even more potent form of fentanyl and can be 1000 times stronger than fentanyl itself.

It takes a lot less of the drug to get the user high and the threat of an overdose is always probable, especially with a drug as potent as this one.

When an overdose occurs, the purity of the drug shuts down the central nervous system and the victim cannot breathe. If the victim of an overdose does not get medical help within 10 minutes or less, there is very little chance of survival.

**HEROIN** - In the 1890's, the concern over morphine addiction was of great concern and a quest to find a nonaddicting narcotic was set. This was an unknowingly foolish quest with no results.

# "Drugs and Beyond"

In 1898, the Bayer Co. commercially introduced heroin which was named from the German word, *heroisch* (meaning, "large," "powerful"). It was a semisynthetic derivative of morphine, being 2 or 3 times as potent.

Today, in North America, heroin is still used as a street drug and in parts of Europe, as a powerful painkiller in medicine.

Heroin is very addictive if a person likes the high they receive from administering the opiates on themselves, although crack and cocaine are even more addictive.

**MORPHINE** - is the chief alkaloid of opium and is used medicinally to dull pain and to cause sleep. It is bitter, colorless or white and is 10 times more potent than opium.

Alkaloids are basic organic substances containing carbon, hydrogen, nitrogen and usually oxygen which generally have pronounced effects on animal organisms. These substances are submitable to unnatural modes of administration. Pure opium, for example, cannot be injected, but morphine, heroin, etc., can.

**METHADONE** - is a synthetic opiate with similar actions and properties to those of all the opiates. It was developed during World War II to replace heroin and morphine and is slightly more potent than the latter and is as addictive as heroin. Twenty years before methadone became the trend or the peoples favorite drug, it was known as dolophine and was used to withdraw people addicted to the opiates.

Opiate users used it when there was short supply of heroin or morphine and to rid withdraw symptoms.

**OTHER OPIATES** - meperidine or pethidine (demerol) is a synthetic derivative of morphine, and hydromorphone (dilaudid) is a semisynthetic derivative.

Demerol is about 10 to 20 percent as potent as morphine and Dilaudid is about 2 times as potent as heroin. Both have long been favorites with users who can persuade physicians to write the prescription.

***Medical Advantages:*** when opiates are taken for medicinal purposes, they can reduce acute pain. Doctors usually prescribe opiates after surgery and for pain relating to illness or injury. They do not cause the pain to go away, but trigger the user into an alternative state of consciousness in which things are experienced differently than they are in a normal state.

A person under the influence of the opiates can still accurately describe the source of the pain and is still aware of the pain, but is no longer concerned or anxious about it and feels detached from it.

Opiates are also used to relieve severe cough and diarrhea, and to prevent and cure colds.

***Illegal Applications:*** opiates and purified opiates prepared for medicinal use, sold for profit.

Fighting against people involved with producing, selling and using these types of drugs is very difficult because of their ingenuousness in concealing, disguising and transporting them.

***Appearance And Methods Of Use:*** All of these narcotics can be taken orally (in most cases having little effect), sniffed through the nasal passages (mild effect) or injected in 3 ways: directly under the skin or "skin-popping", intravenously or "mainlining", and intramuscularly, which has a strong effect. Opium can be smoked, unlike the rest.

***Buprenorphine*** - solution for injection.

***Butorphanol*** - solution for injection.

***Diacetylmorphine (Heroin)*** - is a fine white or brown powder which can be found in three forms: tablet, liquid (linctus), and sealed glass capsules (ampoules). It is usually diluted with other substances and is, in most cases, injected.

***Fentanyl*** - solution for injection or, on the streets, a powder.

***Hydromorphone*** - tablet, suppository or solution for injection.

***Levorphanol*** - tablets or solution for injection.

***Methadone*** - oral concentrate, oral solution, tablets, dispersable tablets, or solution for injection.

***Methylmorphine (Codeine)*** - can be in a/an tablet, capsule, elixir, suppository or solution for injection forms.

***Meperidine (Demerol)*** - an off white tablet, syrup, or solution for injection.

***Morphine*** - in the form of extended-release tablets, oral solution, syrup, suppository or solution for injection.

***Nalbuphine*** - solution for injection.

***Opium*** - dark brown chunks or powder which is usually eaten or smoked, but can be in solution for injection.

***Oxycodone*** - oral solution, tablets or suppositories.

***Oxymorphone*** - suppositories or solution for injection.

# "Drugs and Beyond"

**Pentazocine** - tablets or solution for injection; "Pentazocine and Naloxone" tablets are also available.

**Propoxyphene** - capsules, oral suspension, or tablets.

**Behavioral Characteristics:** drop in grades, sloppy dress, unusual borrowing of money, mood swings, loss of personal possessions (sold to buy drugs), slurred speech, wearing sunglasses (to hide the pupils looking like pinpoints) or the use of visine, weight loss, loss of interest in former goals, difficulty in concentrating, increased illness and change of friends. Also see "Short Term and Long Term Effects" for further evidence of abuse.

**Short Term Effects:** the initial effects depend on a person's mood, environment, amount taken and if the person has any past experience with these types of drugs.
   The effects include: an initial rush of pleasure, stimulation of higher brain centers, depression of the central nervous system, analgesia, relief of severe cough and diarrhea, sleepiness, constipation, nausea and vomiting, dry mouth, drowsiness, moist, cold and blue skin, pinpointed pupils, hallucinations and possible impairment of the respiratory system.

**Long Term Effects:** prolonged use of these drugs produce such effects as: a higher percentage of miscarriages and other birth defects, constipation, decreased sexual drive and menstrual irregularity. When injected, effects can include infections, contraction of the AIDS virus, liver disease, scaring, coma and death.

**NOTE** - when any of this type of drug is taken with other sedatives, death can occur.

**Tolerance and Dependence:** all opiates and opiate substitutes are addictive to some degree and have the potential for abuse. The cravings to take these drugs are strong and can easily overpower the person to the point where everything he/she does involves the drugs.
   Withdrawal symptoms can include a strong craving for the drug, anxiety, a feeling of unpleasantness or discomfort, perspiration, watering eyes, restless broken sleep, runny nose, goose bumps, stomach cramps, diarrhea, yawning, a sense of uneasiness, hot and cold flashes, aching bones and muscles, nausea, vomiting, abdominal cramps, weight loss and low grade fever. The worst of the effects pass within a few days, but can take weeks or months for the body to return to normal again.

For Heroin, when one is addicted, there is hope for the abuser to stop the use of this drug. Other drugs such as Naltrexone are used to slowly reduce the cravings for this drug.

Narceine is a drug which is used to revive an overdosed person. It works by kick-starting the central nervous system giving the victim the ability to breathe and is revived. He/she then can be treated for any further damage which may have been caused.

**Helpful Natural Treatments:** when a person uses the opiates on a regular basis, their body needs special attention. Food is a must and should be taken along with the following:

*Vitamins:* A, B, B complex, B3, B5, B12, C, Sodium ascorbate (buffered vitamin C) and E.

*Minerals:* Calcium, Magnesium (chelated form) and Selenium.

*Aminos:* L-Glutathione, L-Lithium carbonate & L-Phenylalanine.

*Herbs:* Astragalus, Cayenne, Cowslip, Echinacea, Ginseng, Hops, Licorice Root, Lobelia, Milk Thistle, Pau D'Arco, Siberian Ginseng, Golden Seal, Suma, Valerian Root, and Yucca.

*Also:* Acidophilus liquid; a high potency multivitamin; a high potency mineral complex; Bran; GABA (gamma-aminobutyric acid); Red Spearmint. This herb can help to safely alleviate restlessness associated with withdrawal symptoms.

Slowed mental responses &
decreased attention span

Blood shot eyes

Increased acne

Rapid heart beat

Sharpened senses

Decreased short
term memory

Impaired balance

Dry mouth

Lung damage

Poor muscle
coordination

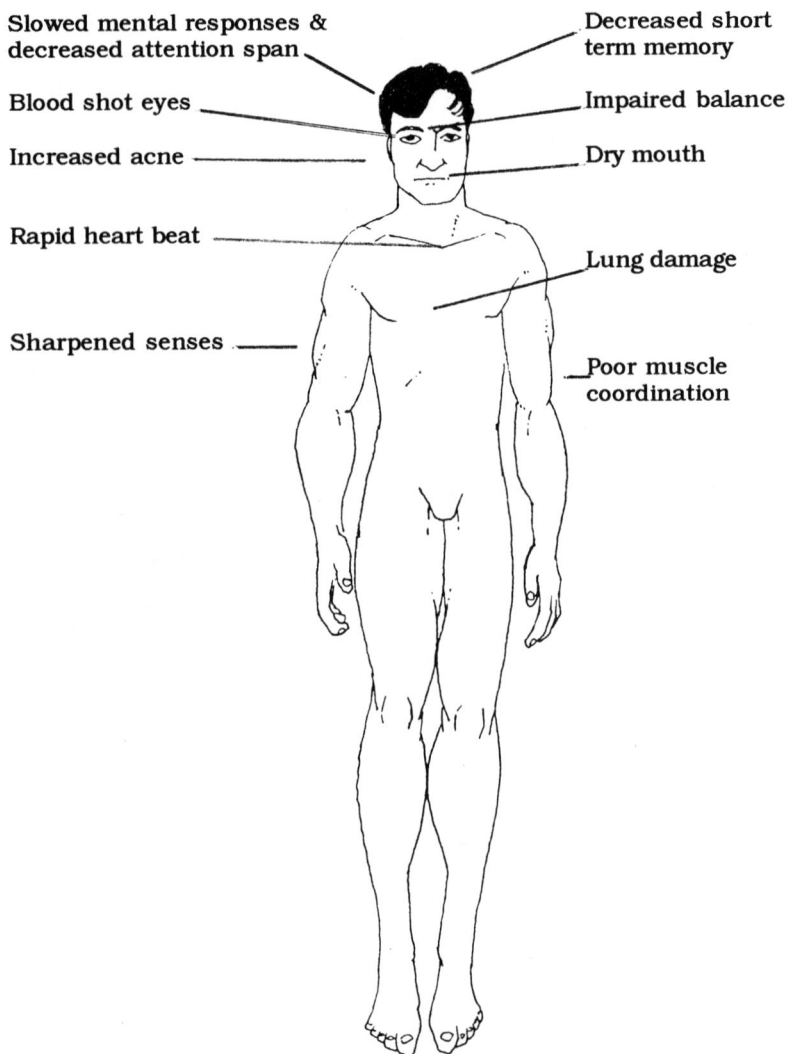

Adverse effects and problem areas associated
with short and long term use of
*Marijuana and its derivatives*

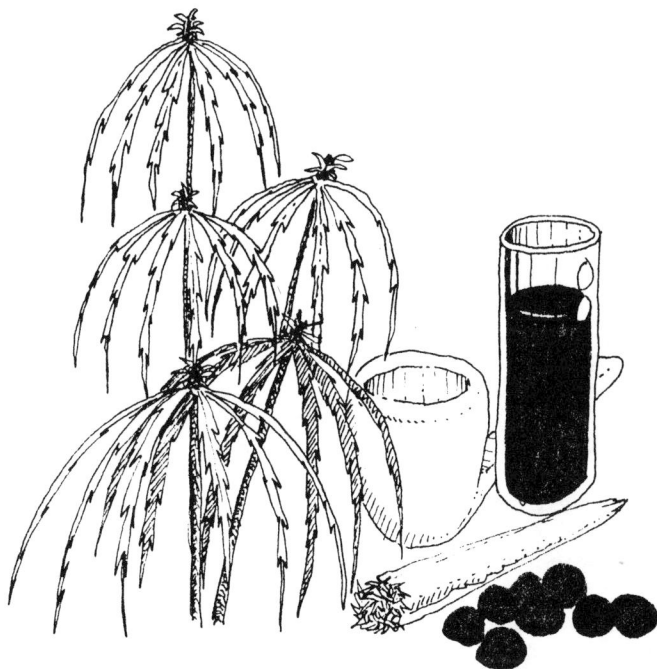

## MARIJUANA

**MARIJUANA** - is an hallucinogenic mood-altering drug which is also known as cannabis. It is from the flowers and leaves of the *Cannabis sativa* plant which possesses euphoric and hallucinogenic effects. THC (delta-9-tetrahydro-cannabinol) is responsible for the effects caused by the use of marijuana and its derivatives.

The weakest form of cannabis is marijuana with up to 7 to 15 percent THC. Hashish has from 10 to 15 percent and hash oil possesses up to 60 percent; although, these figures can vary greatly with different processes of growth and extraction.

Cannabis is usually smoked, but can also be eaten, cooked in food or drank as a tea. The effects caused by smoking cannabis can last from 2 to 3 hours. As a beverage or in food, the effects can last up to 12 hours and is not as intense as the inhalation of smoke.

# "Drugs and Beyond"

In the 1100's, a band of Muslims in Persia and Asia Minor, known as assassins or hashshashins (hemp-eaters), smoked the drug hashish and while under the influence, killed their enemies which is where the word assassination comes from.

Some people believe that the use of cannabis leads to the use of stronger, physically addicting drugs. Although some users of hard drugs started out with marijuana and/or its derivatives, most people explore with the others and usually end up going back to cannabis use.

**Derivatives:** Marijuana - obtained from both the flowering tops and cut and dried leaves and stems; Ganga - comes from dried leaves and flowering shoots; Hashish - a potent resin extracted from the top of the flowering plant; Hash Oil - is what yields from repeated purification of hashish; Honey Oil - is the purest form of the marijuana resins; Weed Oil - is a form of the marijuana resins which is extracted from the entire cannabis sativa plant.

**Brand Names:** unknown.

**Street Names:** Acapulco gold, berkely boo, bhang, boo, brick, bush, charas, Colombian, dope, dugga, duster, ganja, gold, Goma de Mota, goof butt, grass, hash, Hawaiian, hay, hemp, herb, J, Jamaican, jive, joint, key, kif, lid, locoweed, machohina, Marijuana, Maryjane, MJ, mota, muggles, mutah, pod, pot, reefer, roach, rope, sativa, shit, sinsemilla, skunk, smoke, soles, spliff, stick, supergrass, sweet lucy, tea, tocas tea, weed, wheelchair weed, Yerba.

**Medical Advantages:** cannabis can be used: to help asthmatics; in the fight against glaucoma; to rid the body of tumors whether they be benign or malignant; to relieve the nauseating side effect from AIDS and cancer therapy; to help an unsettled stomach common in motion sickness; in the treatment of epilepsy; to relieve back pain and muscle spasms when applied as a poultice; as an antibiotic and disinfectant; to relieve the pain from arthritis, cystic fibrosis and rheumatism when used as a poultice; to kill the herpes virus when used topically; as a lung expectorant (being given the ability to cough up and get rid of phlegm) and cleaner; to help a person sleep better and have a more restful sleep; to help sufferers of emphysema deal with unwanted symptoms and may increase their life expectancy; to deal with stress and migraine headaches; to increase ones appetite which could and has been used to help anorexic people;

to reduce saliva, which can be especially good if a person has to visit the dentist - no cotton balls are needed and limit the use of a suction hose; to raise a persons spirits and/or help a person cope who may have an incurable disease.

***Illegal Applications:*** marijuana and its derivatives illegally grown, processed and sold for profit; purchasing, consuming or inhaling marijuana or its smoke without permission from a figure of authority.

***Appearance And Methods Of Use:*** marijuana and its derivatives can be green, goldish, black, brown, yellowish and everything in between and can be smoked in a hand rolled cigarette (joint) or pipe, cooked in food, eaten raw or made into a tea. Marijuana, in the proper form, can be injected, but is very painful if taken this way and, therefore, is not very common.

***Positive Uses:*** Some of the uses of the *Cannabis sativa* plant are:
hemp (the tough, strong fiber from this plant) used for cloth, ropes and cords; especially, in the past, for the use of a ship' s rigging and the nets needed for fishing. Hemp does not have any effects on the body. It was collected and made into the material needed when the plant decayed and the fiber separated from the stem. This process remains the same today.
Another common use for hemp is hemp paper, known for its longevity and resistance to tearing, which is still used today in Canadian currency and for fine Bibles.
People in China relied on the plant for many other uses than just the hemp fiber. The seeds were one of the grains of early China along with rice, barley, millet, and soybeans. The seeds were ground into meal, roasted whole or cooked in porridge. Sacrificial vessels filled with hemp seed and other grains were placed into ancient tombs of China for the afterlife.
The oil from the plant was also used by the Chinese civilized nations. Pressed seeds produced almost 20 percent oil by weight. Similar to linseed oil, it was used for cooking, to fuel lamps, for lubrication and as a base in paints, varnish and soap making. When the process of pressing for oil extraction was completed, about 10 percent oil and 30 percent protein still remained which was used as a nutritious feed for domesticated animals.
Today, it could be one of the options to be considered to fuel transportation without causing the pollution and to make paper products which could save the rain forests.

# "Drugs and Beyond"

**Behavioral Characteristics:** unusual borrowing of money, loss of personal possessions (sold to buy drugs), drop in grades, sloppy dress, burn holes in clothes, mood swings, constant cough, increased illness, use of candles and incense, cold room (frequent airing out), change of friends, wearing sunglasses or the use of visine (to hide the redness of the eyes), bent paper clips (used to hold a marijuana cigarette), seeds in pockets of clothing, possible weight gain due to constant consumption of junk food and pop or other flavored beverages taken to satisfy the bodies need for food when the user is high, loss of interest in former goals, difficulty in concentrating, strange paraphernalia in or around the house or property of the user, and slurred speech. Also see "Short Term and Long Term Effects" for further evidence of abuse.

**Short Term Effects:** When taken, one becomes relaxed, some people become talkative and others become quiet and withdrawn, senses feel sharper, ordinary objects take on special meaning, judging distance and passage of time becomes difficult, attention span and concentration may be reduced, remembering things that have just happened becomes difficult, simple tasks become a challenge, impaired balance, rapid heartbeat (as much as a 50 percent increase, depending on the potency), red eyes, increased appetite, dry mouth and throat, drowsiness, confusion and anxiety.

When higher doses are taken, the user may have mild hallucinations and feelings of panic. These effects disappear as the drugs effects ware off.

Poor muscle coordination and drowsiness make it hazardous to drive any vehicle and the inability to use machinery properly, thus, safety may cause a threat to the user and others around him or her.

**Long Term Effects:** A marijuana cigarette contains almost four times the amount of tar as a tobacco cigarette and, therefore, has a much higher risk of damaging the lungs which increases the chances of contracting lung cancer and other related diseases.

Prolonged cannabis use may result in slowed mental responses, reduced drive, inability to do complex tasks, communication skills are lessened, failure to make long term plans and neglect of personal appearance. It is not known if cannabis use causes birth defects, but use during pregnancy is not recommended.

**NOTE** - marijuana is occasionally contaminated with animal droppings containing Salmonella bacteria either at the time of drying or during storage.

This organism, which is not destroyed by drying, can cause diarrhea, abdominal pain and fever. A herbicide called paraquat, which is used by the government to destroy marijuana crops, poses another threat to one's health.

**Tolerance and Dependence:** there is no physical dependence developed through the use of marijuana. Slight psychological dependence and tolerance are built to marijuana.

### Helpful Natural Treatments:

*Vitamins:* A, B complex, B3, B5, B12, C, Sodium ascorbate (buffered vitamin C) and E.

*Minerals:* Calcium, Magnesium (chelated form) and Selenium.

*Aminos:* L-Glutathione, L-Lithium carbonate & L-Phenylalanine.

*Herbs:* Astragalus, Cayenne, Cowslip, Echinacea, Ginseng, Hops, Licorice Root, Lobelia, Milk Thistle, Pau D'Arco, Siberian Ginseng, Golden Seal, Suma, Valerian Root, and Yucca.

Whole Foods: Citrus fruit and green leafy vegetables.

*Also:* a high potency multivitamin; a high potency mineral complex; GABA (gamma-aminobutyric acid).

# "Drugs and Beyond"

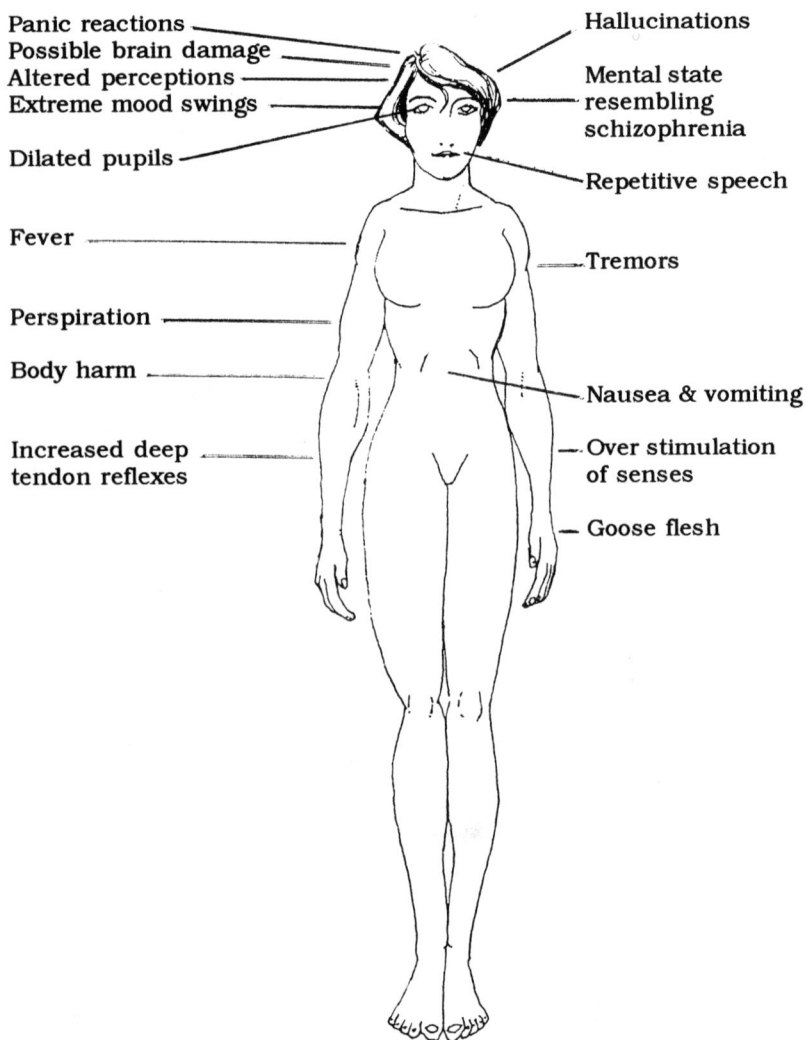

Panic reactions
Possible brain damage
Altered perceptions
Extreme mood swings

Dilated pupils

Fever

Perspiration

Body harm

Increased deep
tendon reflexes

Hallucinations

Mental state
resembling
schizophrenia

Repetitive speech

Tremors

Nausea & vomiting

Over stimulation
of senses

Goose flesh

Adverse effects and problem areas associated
with short and long term use of
## Psychedelics (hallucinogens)

## PSYCHEDELICS and HALLUCINOGENS

**HALLUCINOGENS** - substances which excite the brain, causing hallucination, mood change, mistakes in judgments, loss in sense of self; increased pulse, temperature and blood pressure along with widened pupils. Use of hallucinogens may lead to habit, as well as possible depression or short-term insanity if abused.

**PSYCHEDELICS** - drugs or substances having an effect of seeming to expand consciousness and perception.

The following details apply for all the hallucinogens that follow, although some may appear to be more prevalent with specific drugs.

These drugs produce mixed and intense feelings characterized by that of being relaxed and peaceful, yet anxious and tense; feelings of happiness and sadness at the same time.

This state is described as being multipotential. This simply means that the person can take many paths out of this state.

People who are fearful and anxious may start to panic for a short time and become almost psychotic, but as the drugs effects ware off, so do the extreme feelings. While a person is in this panic state, the best way a person can help is simply to talk to the person calmly and keep him/her in touch with reality.

Those who open themselves up to the experience, resolve the intense feelings and may leave the experience with deep personal insights, religious union and/or increased creative abilities.

While amidst the experience, people may see value and meaning in things, contrary to their normal conscious state in which they may see the same things as being trivial.

Psychiatrists believe that these feelings resemble those of a person just before becoming psychotic or schizophrenic, although it is claimed that cocaine and amphetamines may be better representatives of these disorders.

There is the risk of prolonged depression and/or anxiety following the use of one of the psychedelic drugs. People with psychological problems run the risk of possible prolonged psychotic states associated with these types of drugs.

These drugs commonly cause what is known as a "flashback." During a flashback, the drug's effects recur spontaneously which can involve either the visual hallucinations or any other sensory

# "Drugs and Beyond"

element of the original experience even though the person may not have used the drug for weeks or even months. A flashback is possible to occur after just one use, but is more likely to occur in regular users. The episodes are, in most cases, brief, lasting only a few minutes or seconds.

Deaths from hallucinogen overdose have not been reported with the exception of the phenylisopropylamines because of their molecular structure resembling that of the amphetamines. However, these drugs have been implicated in suicides, accidental deaths, murders and self-inflicted wounds. When used by expectant mothers, birth defects and/or miscarriages have been noted.

**Behavioral actions and characteristics** include the following: possible poor hygiene, one feels happy and sad at the same time; emotional swings, dilated pupils, strange behavior not typical of the person under normal conditions, suspiciousness, nausea and vomiting, unusual hilarity, increased pulse and blood pressure,

**If there is suspicion of use**, the following items are what to look for which will most likely have been hidden in a place of privacy such as, in a bedroom, in clothing, behind light switch covers or pictures, or in a bathroom (especially in the tank of the toilet): capsules or pills in various colors, sizes, and shapes; rolling papers; pieces or clumps of aluminum foil; small or medium size plastic sandwich or freezer bags.

**Less commonly used items are**: syringes, tubes (such as plastic, metal or wooden straws) or a folded matchbook or paper in the shape of a scoop which are used to snort the drugs. Not all items and paraphernalia can be listed because of the ingenuousness of substance abusers.

**Effects which are due to the actions of these types of drugs are:** exhaustion with possible surges of energy, fever, an increase in acne, dilated pupils, rapid pulse, nausea and vomiting, loss of appetite, tremors, increased and quickened deep tendon reflexes, insomnia, relaxation, anxiety, tension, possibility of convulsions, repetitive speech, useless activities (these may include picking at the skin for hours on end, pacing the floor, constant movement of the legs and/or arms, etc.), panic and anxiety states may occur, a toxic delirium, perspiration, goose flesh, depression after the drugs effects have worn off, suicidal tendencies during the "trip", blurred vision, fear of going crazy, pondering over detail, clumsiness which may lead to accidental death, prolonged psychotic breaks, chronic brain syndromes, schizophrenic episodes, intensified emotional activity, relative loss of time, dreamy states, extreme sensitivity to stimuli, hallucinations, euphoria and rarely, violence to others and to self.

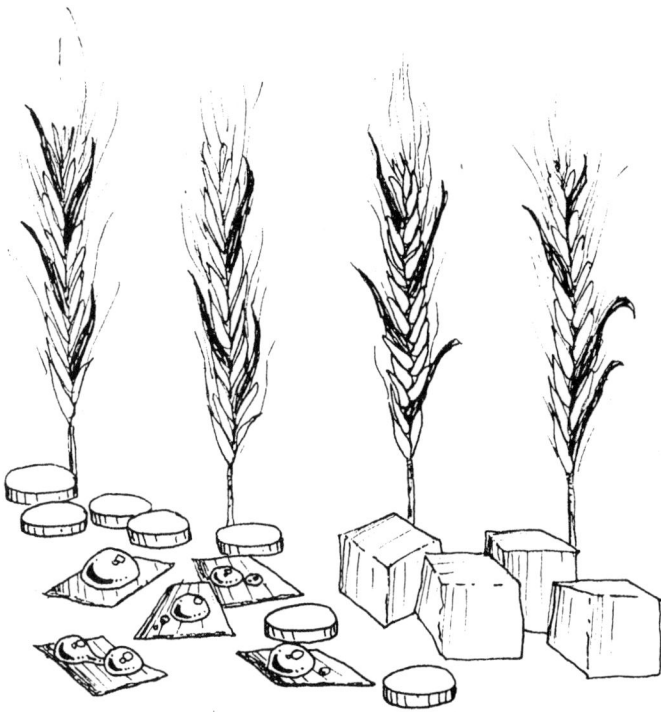

## LSD-25 (d - lysergic acid diethylamide, or "acid") -

is a derivative of an acid extracted from the rye grain fungus, ergot. It is colorless, tasteless, and odorless with a potency being compared to one ounce having the ability to be divided into 300, 000 doses. It is derived from the rye grain fungus (Claviceps purpurea), which has been used for centuries to aid childbirth and is described in the earliest botanical literature.

All naturally occurring hallucinogens (except THC) are alkaloids. There are many ergot alkaloids and among them is the lysergic amide series, of which the twenty-fifth preparation (LSD-25) was tested.

At first, it was discovered accidentally and later by design, by a 37 year old Swiss chemist at Sandoz Pharmaceutical labs in Basel. He, Dr. Albert Hofmann, absorbed a drop of the solution on his finger and began to notice that reality was pleasant and was almost like a fairy-tale. He reported "a laboratory intoxication" and a few days later, on April 19, deliberately swallowed some more, beginning with the moderate amount of 250 micrograms, or 25 millionths of a gram.

# "Drugs and Beyond"

There is no other substance which produces effects with such a small dose, and Hofmann unknowingly began "tripping out." On his way home, riding his bicycle, he thought he was going insane, but it was only the temporary effects of the drug. Further tests by volunteers proved psychic potential, but because of interruptions caused by the war, it took four years for the news to reach the medical world.

The psychiatric profession immediately grabbed this new drug, as did Cold War military - intelligence specialists.

The U.S. Army tested it as an incapacitating agent in warfare and as means of reversing the effects of brainwashing on Korean War POWs.

LSD was first given to mental patients in sterile hospital rooms and clinics by doctors who followed contemporary standards of maximum objectivity and did not, themselves, take the drug. Schizophrenics and the psychotic would quite often have bad trips, but some had gained temporary insight into their illness.

Ergot poisoning (a disease in rye and other cereals in which the grains are replaced by blackish fungous growths) may have been a significant factor in the Salem witch trials. Outbreaks occurred from time to time in European villages, as recently as 1951, where rye bread was a main food staple. The people affected with the ergot poisoning would see others, or sometimes even themselves, as strange beasts or distorted beings; thought to be witches.

This was complicated further when these supposed witches would make love potions from an assortment of herbs. One common herb used in these potions was mandrake (discussed later in this book) which would make its users feel that they were flying. At the same time, an ecstatic feeling would power over them and some had been noted trying to please themselves with a broom, sometimes brooms.

These visions soon gave way to the belief that the people seen were possessed and evil, therefore, they must be witches and were usually killed.

**Derivatives:** ergot fungus.

**Brand Names:** LSD-25.

**Street Names:** acid, barrels, blotter, blue cap, blue cheer, blue dots, California Sunshine, camel, candles, cherry top, Cube-D, dragon, king tut, Lucy in the sky with diamonds, man, micro dots, Mr. Natural, orange sunshine, owsleys, owsley's orange sunshine, paper acid, purple haze, 25, white lightning, wedges, wedgies, window panes, zigzag man.

**Medical Advantages:** may possess the ability to treat patients suffering from personality disorders such as anorexia, obsessive-compulsive disorders and depression. To prove this, the Swiss government licensed a group of psychiatrists to use the drug. 100 to 200 microgram doses of LSD (which differs from the psychedelic strength of 500 micrograms) were being administered to patients to enhance the therapeutic process by making repressed memories and feeling more accessible. The results were positive and up to date, there are some 150 documented cases on the efficiency of LSD in conjunction to psychotherapy.

**Illegal Applications:** the production, selling, purchasing or consuming LSD in any form without authorization from proper authorities.

**Appearance And Methods Of Use:** taken orally as colored drops on blotting paper or the solution can be put into anything which can be consumed; a common way being sugar cubes. Also in tablet, capsule and liquid forms. The tablets are found in an arrange of colors, but the more common are orange and blue.

**Short Term Effects:** felt within 1 hour and lasting up to 18 hours. The users perceptions are altered, thinking and concentration become difficult, short-term memory is impaired and a person may have extreme mood swings.

**Long Term Effects:** possibility of brain damage and, if the dose is too high, a possible permanent psychotic or schizophrenic state may occur.

**Tolerance and Dependence:** LSD is not addictive. Users of LSD find that they need more of the drug to get the same effect as their previous trip. With daily use, and as larger doses are taken, they won't have any different effect on a person's feelings or mind, but will continue the damaging effects on the body. LSD was a popular drug in the 1960s and although it is less widely used today, it is still a potent drug whose dangerous side effects are not completely understood.

**Helpful Natural Treatments:**

*Vitamins:* A, B, B complex, B3, B5, B12, C, Sodium ascorbate (buffered vitamin C) and E.

*Minerals:* Calcium, Magnesium (chelated form) and Selenium.

*Aminos:* L-Glutathione, L-Lithium carbonate & L-Phenylalanine.

*Herbs:* Astragalus, Cowslip, Echinacea, Hops, Licorice Root, Lobelia, Siberian Ginseng, Golden Seal, Valerian Root, and Yucca.

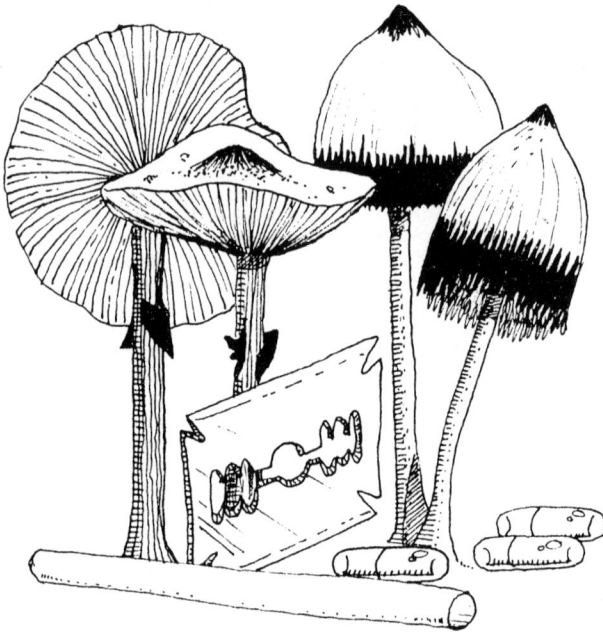

## MAGIC MUSHROOMS

**Magic Mushrooms** - Mushrooms or toadstools are of the family of fungi. People usually give the name "mushroom" to the kind of fungi that can be eaten and "toadstool" to those that are poisonous.

*Amanita muscaria* or *fly agaric mushroom*, is a type of mushroom in which muscimole is responsible for its effects. It grows in northern temperate zones of North America and in parts of Europe and Asia; the most potent variety found in Siberia.

*Amanita pantherina* is another variety which is similar in appearance to Amanita muscaria, but is somewhat stronger in its effects.

The effects of the drug begin 15 minutes to 1 1/2 hours after ingestion. The psychedelic effects peak after 2 to 2 1/2 hours and slowly decrease thereafter, with the effects lasting a total of about 8 hours.

The effects and duration of effects can vary depending on the type of mushroom and amount taken.

Dizziness or drowsiness, loss of coordination, numbness of the legs and the possibility of nausea are the initial reactions. These soon give way to dreamy visual hallucinations, especially size distortion, a growing euphoria, mental clarity in which everything seems to be more alive, and visions of bright colors and patterns similar to those seen on virtual reality programs. Physical strength and energy may increase before the end of the trip which consists of the user falling into a deep sleep.

Siberian tribesmen would eat the Amanita muscaria mushrooms in intervals. They would start by eating a small amount of one mushroom, increasing their intake slowly and in half-hour intervals, but would not exceed three mushrooms. The continuation of the "high" could be achieved by drinking their own urine or the urine of another mushroom eater. Three or four successive urination's still retained some of the original potency of the fungi, because muscimol is unchanged by the digestion process and is simply discarded by the body through the urine. Siberian women were excluded from such practices, other than premoistening them before they were ingested by the men.

**Psilocybin** and **psilocin** are psychedelic agents found in the Mexican magic mushroom. These mushrooms have been used throughout Central America for many years for religious and sacramental purposes.

The mushrooms are eaten raw and are only 1 percent as potent as LSD. When the mushrooms are consumed, the body changes psilocybin into psilocin, which is 1.4 times stronger than psylocybin.

The effects are very similar to those of LSD, but do not last as long; between 2 and 8 hours.

**Derivatives:** psilocybin, psilocin, muscimole.

**Brand Names:** none.

**Street Names:** magic mushrooms, shrooms, silly putty.

**Medical Advantages:** may help to give a better understanding of psychiatric disorders and can aid in childbirth as a painkiller and to dilate the uterus.

**Illegal Applications:** the growing, cultivation, consuming, selling and purchasing magic mushrooms without authorization from proper authorities.

# "Drugs and Beyond"

**Appearance And Methods Of Use:** can be taken orally in natural form (fresh or dried), as a tea, as a capsule containing powder of any color, by snorting, or smoked with another medium such as marijuana.

**Short Term Effects:** altered perceptions, relaxation, fatigue and sometimes laughter. Larger doses produce abdominal discomfort, numbness, sweating and dizziness.

**Long Term Effects:** possible memory loss and brain damage although it is very minimal.

### Helpful Natural Treatments:

*Vitamins:* A, B complex, B3, B5, B9, B12, C, Sodium ascorbate (buffered vitamin C) and E.

*Minerals:* Calcium, Magnesium (chelated form) and Selenium.

*Aminos:* L-Glutathione, L-Lithium carbonate & L-Phenylalanine.

*Herbs:* Astragalus, Cayenne, Cowslip, Echinacea, Ginseng, Hops, Licorice Root, Lobelia, Milk Thistle, Pau D'Arco, Siberian Ginseng, Golden Seal, Suma, Valerian Root, and Yucca.

*Also:* a high potency multivitamin; a high potency mineral complex; GABA (gamma-aminobutyric acid).

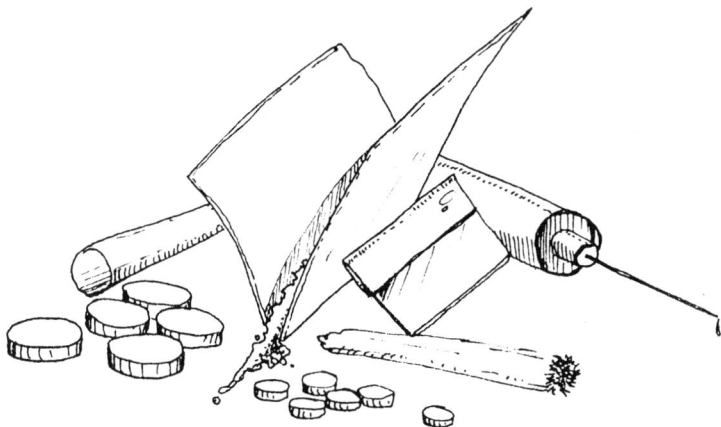

## PHENCYCLIDINE

***Phencyclidine (1-[1-phenylcyclohexyl] piperidine HCL)*** - is of the class of mind-altering drugs known as dissociatives or arylcyclohexylamines and, although it is classified here as a psychedelic or an hallucinogen, it is pharmacologically and behaviorally distinct from the rest.

It is an anesthetic and a stable solid readily soluble in water or ethanol. Being an anesthetic means that when it is taken, the person does not feel pain. This may result in the user causing himself/herself bodily harm by falling down stairs, burning oneself, getting a cut, etc. which will not be felt until the high has worn off.

After being developed in the late 1950's, interest was stirred for its use as a dissociative anesthetic. In clinical trials, patients who were to have surgery were anesthetized with PCP and felt dissociated from their surroundings. Analgesia and some amnesia was noted, but with no significant cardiovascular or respiratory depression. The problems associated with the drug were mild to extreme disorientation, hallucinations, delirium, agitation and manic excitation. For this reason, in 1965, human studies were discontinued.

# "Drugs and Beyond"

There are over 30 phencyclidine analogs developed through minor changes in the manufacturing process. Some of the more popular street preparations are ketamine, PCE, PCPy, PHP, TCP and TPCP.

Ketamine was the most common anesthetic used during the Vietnam War. It is a liquid when manufactured, but on the streets can be bought in powder, pill or capsule forms or bought soaked in marijuana, parsley or tobacco. Users describe it as being an out of this world, dreamlike state, but problems associated with these drugs can be severe.

Some problems associated with these analogs are that they can contain high levels of contaminants which can be very harmful to the user's system. Also they are sometimes combined with other abused drugs such as stimulants, depressants, and other hallucinogens, which can have extremely harmful effects.

**Derivatives:** there are over 30 derivatives of phencyclidine. The more common are: Ketamine, PC, PCC, PCE, PCPy, PHP, TCP, TPCP.

**Brand Names:** Sernyl, Sernylan, Synalar. Some analogs' names are Ketamine or Ketalar, PCE (N-ethyl-1-phenylcyclohexylamine), TCP or TPCP (1-[1-(2-thienyl)-cyclohexyl] piperidine), PCPy and PHP (1-[1-phenylcyclohexyl] pyrrolidine).

**Street Names:** angel dust, crystal, cyclone, DOA (**D**ead **O**n **A**rrival or **D**ust **O**f **A**ngels), dummy dust, dust, elephant, embalming fluid, goon, hog, horse tranquilizer, itog, killer weed, krystal, love boat, mint, mintweed, monkey dust, ozone, **P**ea**C**e **P**ill, PCE, PCP, PCPy, peace, PHP, rocket fuel, scuffle, sherman, supergrass, superkool, superpot, surfer, T, tac, TCP, tic tac, TPCP, Tran Q, tranq, weed.

**Medical Advantages:** a small peptide in the brain has been found to bind to one PCP receptor and produce PCP like effects in animals. This could mean that the drug acts on neuronal systems already active in the brain. This has led to the development of PCP antagonists and antibodies to decrease the drug's toxicity in animals. Further experimentation with these substances may lead to useful therapeutic agents for PCP users in psychotic episodes.

**Illegal Applications:** although it is a very complex drug, pharmacologically, it is easily synthesized and is done so in basement -, garage -, van -, etc., type laboratories and is then sold for profit.

It is taken illicitly for its overwhelming properties which gives the user: feelings of strength, power, invulnerability, and a numbing effect on the mind which often gives the user feelings of anger, rage, and an absence of unpleasant memories. Because of the lower cost of a high, cocaine addicts have been known to use PCP as a substitute.

**Appearance And Methods Of Use:** a white, crystalline powder containing the drug at 50 to 100 percent strength is usually mixed with leafy material and smoked. Its analogs contain a high level of contaminants which can change the color and consistency from a tan to a brown and from a powder to a gummy mass.

Phencyclidine and its analogs can be taken orally (as a pill or tablet which can be found in a variety of colors), by injection, by snorting, or by inhalation from a cigarette which has been sprinkled (dusted) with the powder form.

**Behavioral Characteristics:** signs to look for if there is suspicion of abuse are: amnesia, delusions, dissociations, dry and red skin, enlarged pupils, excitement, and a continuous involuntary movement of the eyes.

Others signs are: agitation, anxiety, irregular heartbeat, catalepsy, catatonia, coma, convulsions, death, perspiration, disorganization, inability to control bowel movements, euphoria, excitement, fever, flushing, hyperreflexia, hypersalivation, hypertensive, hyporeflexia, irritability, opisthotonos, psychosis, the muscles are hard, tense or stiff, repetitive behavior, tactile hallucinations, violence and visual hallucinations.

Most withdrawal signs are similar to those of a major depression and include: anorexia, decreased sexual desire, depression, insomnia and cravings for the drug.

**Short Term Effects:** (taken in low doses; 5 mg.) produces excitement, muscle stiffness and lack of coordination, slurred speech, drowsiness, confusion and general numbness of the extremities, nausea, profuse sweating, increased heart rate is possible, sense of separation from one's surroundings, difficulties in concentration and communicating and flushing of the skin; sensations of distortions of time, space, body image and may become highly confused. With higher doses, one may also become, or it may cause paranoid, terrified, either aggressive or passive, drooling, vomiting, stupor or coma; some, but not all, experience a state of extreme euphoria.

**Long Term Effects:** speech impediments, anxiety, memory loss, depression, decreased respiration, body stiffness or tension, epileptic seizures, coma and possibly death if not treated promptly. Also, it acts like an analgesic. With this reduction or loss of the ability to feel pain, injury to oneself can be life threatening, if not fatal due to cuts, bruising or broken bones which are not usually noticed or felt until the drug's effects have worn off.

**Tolerance and Dependence:** tolerance is built and dependence is possible with habitual use of phencyclidine. Different effects may be produced each time the drug is used with serious short and long term effects varying from person to person.

Kainic acid may be an important factor in controlling the potency of this drug. Depending on the amount given, it has the ability to increase or decrease the effects of this drug.

### Helpful Natural Treatments:

*Vitamins:* A, B complex, B3, B5, B12, C, Sodium ascorbate (buffered vitamin C) and E.

*Minerals:* Calcium, Magnesium (chelated form) and Selenium.

*Aminos:* L-Glutathione, L-Lithium carbonate & L-Phenylalanine.

*Herbs:* Astragalus, Cayenne, Cowslip, Echinacea, Ginseng, Hops, Licorice Root, Lobelia, Milk Thistle, Pau D'Arco, Siberian Ginseng, Golden Seal, Suma, Valerian Root, and Yucca.

*Also:* Acidophilus liquid; a high potency multivitamin; a high potency mineral complex; Bran; GABA (gamma-aminobutyric acid).

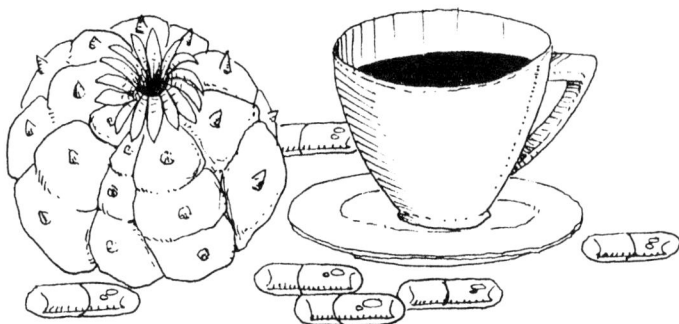

# PEYOTE/MESCALINE

**Peyote** - (Lophophora williamsii) is a gray-green spineless cactus with a small dome-shaped head having tufts of whitish hair and a long root shaped like a carrot. The cacti are found in clusters whose roots are interconnected beneath the ground. The plant contains over 50 alkaloids, but the psychoactive mescaline is found at the top. When cut off and dried, the grooved tops (peyote or mescal buttons) keep their potency for a long period of time, though are more potent when eaten fresh.

**Mescaline** - (3, 4, 5 - trimethoxyphenylethylamine) is an indole, like the majority of psychedelics, but is structurally related to the adrenal hormones and to the synthetic stimulant methamphetamine; which are all very active in the peripheral nervous system. Mescaline comes on over a period of several hours and lasts for 8 to 12. When synthetic mescaline is used, the nausea-provoking effects are greatly reduced, if not entirely eliminated, as compared to peyote itself. The visual effects are what made it most interesting to the European explorers in the early stages of its use in the late 1800's.

**Derivatives:** mescaline.

**Brand Name:** mescaline.

# "Drugs and Beyond"

**Street Names:** big chief, buttons, cactus, mesc, mescal, mescaline, peyote.

**Medical Advantages:** antibiotic properties - very effective against many strains of bacteria and can be used if the bacteria causing the problem are penicillin-resistant.

Psychotherapeutic properties - can be used to help cure alcoholism and other drug addictions. It can also aid in relieving distress and acute depression along with other such problems.

Antiseptic properties - can be used to clean open wounds and cuts. When used in this manner, it can help the healing process and will create a strong, flexible scab that draws the skin tissues together which can make a seal better than stitches.

A home remedy has been used by native people for centuries with positive effects against arthritis, rheumatism, pleurisy, common flu and colds, nerve spasms and paralysis, sciatica, blindness, hearing disorders, and to help in the relief of pain from broken bones and childbirth.

A common misconception is that peyote contains chemicals which will damage chromosomes. A study was done on the "Effects of Peyote on Human Chromosomes" by David Dorrance, MD (Journal of the American Medical Association, 1975 - Vol. 234, No. 3, Oct.) which concluded that "...no significant chromosomal aberrations were apparent among the peyote - and non-peyote - using Huichol Indians."

**Illegal Applications:** mescaline is rarely used as a street drug, but when encountered on the street, it is always in the form of mescaline sulphate, a white crystal packed in a large capsule. Large gelatin capsules filled with brownish peyote bits are occasionally seen. Dried peyote buttons are also rarely seen. The mescaline taker may experience various imaginary or hallucinatory effects while under the drug's influence. Bold and beautiful colors and lights, the transformation of ones companions and oneself into strange beasts or abstract forms, the illusions of weightlessness, even total freedom from the body are some of these effects. But the underlying similarity in the reports of most users is: a feeling of exaltation and a certainty that the vision is fraught with spiritual significance.

**Appearance And Methods Of Use:** the peyote plant is usually eaten, though can be drank as a beverage when mixed with another liquid or liquids.

It takes several hours to chew the buttons, when the whitish hair is removed, because of the toughness and the nausea - provoking bitterness. It can also be ground up into a powder and eaten with honey, drank with fruit juice or as a tea, but it still takes a lot to get it down.

One should be cautious because compounds sold as mescaline on the street may not be mescaline at all. LSD or one of the mescaline derivatives are quite often used as substitutes. This means that users should be very careful because higher doses of these substitutes may be very dangerous and could result in death.

**Short Term Effects:** nausea, body heaviness and possibility of minor muscle spasms of the legs. Can alters one's perception, mood, short-term memory and concentration. Pupils dilate and a person runs the risk of fever, nausea and vomiting.

**Long Term Effects:** it is possible that regular consumption of peyote could be psychologically damaging. A dose of 350-500 mg. will produce increased heart rate and blood pressure, dilated pupils and elevated body temperature. Toxic doses may produce convulsions, and death due to respiratory depression.

**Tolerance and Dependence:** drugs can contain poisonous alkaloids such as strychnine which can be very harmful or fatal. Peyote contains no such alkaloids and is not harmful in the long term, unless taken in toxic levels. For this reason, no deaths have ever been attributed to the use of peyote and no physical or psychological dependence have been reported. Cross-tolerance to both psilocybin and LSD exist and, therefore, since LSD and psilocybin work on serotonin and not adrenalin, it is suspected that mescaline does the same.

### Helpful Natural Treatments:

*Vitamins:* A, B complex, B3, B5, B9, B12, C, Sodium ascorbate (buffered vitamin C) and E.

*Minerals:* Calcium, Magnesium (chelated form) and Selenium.

*Aminos:* L-Glutathione, L-Lithium carbonate & L-Phenylalanine.

*Herbs:* Astragalus, Cayenne, Cowslip, Echinacea, Ginseng, Hops, Licorice Root, Lobelia, Milk Thistle, Pau D'Arco, Siberian Ginseng, Golden Seal, Suma, Valerian Root, and Yucca.

*Also:* a high potency multivitamin; a high potency mineral complex; GABA (gamma-aminobutyric acid).

# "Drugs and Beyond"

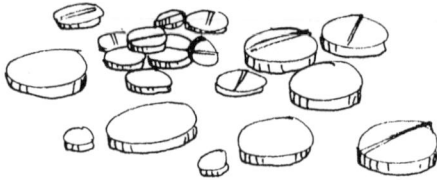

## Methoxylated Amphetamines, Psychomimetic Amphetamines or Phenylisopropylamines

The following are amphetamine analogs of mescaline and make up a group that contains more than a thousand different related chemical substances, of which only a few have been experimented with by man. They all fit into the same family or subgroup of amphetamine which produce effects of both hallucinogens and methamphetamine. These drugs have chemical similarities to amphetamine and mescaline and effects similar amphetamines at low doses and mescaline or LSD at high doses. Both hallucinogens and amphetamines can be produced from these derivatives, although in some cases, molecular substitutions make it impossible.

The more common of these are:

**DOB** (4-bromo-2,5-dimethoxyamphetamine)

**DOE** (2,5-dimethoxy-4-methylamphetamine)

**DOET** (2,5-dimethoxy-4-ethylamphetamine)

**DOM** or **STP** (2,5-dimethoxy-4-methylamphetamine)

**MDA** (methylenedioxyamphetamine)

**MDE** or **MDEA** (N-monoethyl methylenedioxymethamphetamine)

**MDMA** (3,4-methylenedioxymethamphetamine

**MMDA** (3-methoxy-4,5-methylenedioxyamphetamine)

**TMA** (3,4,5-trimethoxyamphetamine).

As doses are increased to enhance the effects, they begin to differ from those of mescaline by producing hyperactivity and hyperexcitability, with accompanying disturbances of body function; closely resembling those of amphetamines and hallucinations similar to LSD. Because of the toxicity of these drugs, safety is definitely reduced and overdoses are more prevalent, although, in most cases deaths have not been reported.

Tremors, that may lead to convulsive movements and which leave the user worn out, are set on by high doses. These high doses and symptoms of high doses may lead to death if not treated.

**NOTE:** If these signs are noticed, contact a doctor immediately!

Along with the aspect of safety, compounds sold as mescaline on the street may not be mescaline at all. LSD or one of the mescaline derivatives are quite often used as substitutes. This means that users should be very careful because higher doses of these substitutes may be very dangerous and could result in death.

Although these drugs are on the Schedule 1 list, they are still being experimented with for possible medical uses. Some of which may help give psychiatric therapy a better understanding why schizophrenia and other psychiatric disorders exist and what people affected with these disorders are feeling, which could lead to a permanent cure.

Others have an added benefit to therapy in respects to their properties of giving a person the ability to share painful emotional issues. This, in turn, will allow them to deal with these issues and become a (using this word loosely) "normal" member of society.

Illicit use of these drugs has not become more prevalent, society is just becoming more aware of the problems associated with these drugs and the ease of accessibility.

These drugs are found on the street in pill or capsule forms of varying colors and have the potential to bring a person closer to ones-self and to others, depending on the amount used. Yet, if taken in higher doses, they have the potential to make a person very irritable, aggressive and withdrawn from others around him or her. Also, if taken in too high of doses, convulsions and agitation are possible, which could lead to death, although this is not common.

The degree of physical or psychological dependence is not known, but if the user takes a liking to the effects brought on by these drugs, the chance of psychological dependence will most certainly be a factor and increase the risk.

Another variable for dependence is why the person is using these drugs. If they are taken in low doses for their amphetaminelike properties, dependence will be at a higher risk. Tolerance is developed quickly with these drugs, which will increase health risks involved as doses are increased to produce effects of previous use.

# "Drugs and Beyond"

A person who uses any of the drugs listed below, on a regular basis, should replenish their body with the following. Some of these are depleted and must be replaced to help the body to continue functioning normally. Others are listed to produce a more rapid recovery.

### Helpful Natural Treatments:

*Vitamins:* A, B complex, B3, B5, B12, C, Sodium ascorbate (buffered vitamin C) and E.

*Minerals:* Calcium, Magnesium (chelated form) and Selenium.

*Aminos:* L-Glutathione, L-Lithium carbonate & L-Phenylalanine.

*Foods:* dark green leaves, flax, hemp seed, pumpkin seed, soy bean and walnut.

*Herbs:* Astragalus, Cayenne, Cowslip, Echinacea, Ginseng, Hops, Licorice Root, Lobelia, Milk Thistle, Pau D'Arco, Siberian Ginseng, Golden Seal, Suma, Valerian Root, and Yucca.

*Also:* a high potency multivitamin; a high potency mineral complex; GABA (gamma-aminobutyric acid); Red Spearmint. This herb can help to safely alleviate restlessness associated with withdrawal symptoms.

Some of the specific drugs listed above are described further below.

## DOM (STP) 2,5-dimethoxy-4-methylamphetamine - is
about 100 times as potent as mescaline, but only 1/3 the potency of LSD. When sold on the street in pill form, it is found to be in rather high doses, some as high as 10 mg. These high doses produce a rather long duration of effects, up to days at a time.

DOM is quite often substituted for mescaline and is the most potent form of the phenylisopropylamines.

The acronym, STP, is used in the street to describe, not only the drug, but the effects brought on by the use of this drug; Super-Terrific Psychedelic or Serenity, Tranquillity and Peace.

At low doses, DOM produces amphetaminelike effects and at high doses, produces LSDlike effects. A dose of 1 to 3 mg. will bring on euphoria similar to that of amphetamine and a dose of 3 to 5 mg. will result in 6 to 8 hours of hallucinations similar to LSD. There is the possibility that, when taken in doses of 10 mg. or more, the effects may last for a day or more.

## MDA (3-methoxy-4,5-methylenedioxyamphetamine) -
called the love pill, MDA was first synthesized in the 1930's when the popularity of mescaline and related mescaline amphetamine compounds was prevalent.

Many users focus on their own lives and personalities rather than what is going on around them when under the influence of MDA.

**Short Term Effects:** the trip lasts about 8 hours and produces such effects as intense feelings, little perceptual changes with an increased insight into things which may seem trivial to others or the user under normal conditions, heightened empathy with others, agitation, convulsions, enhanced mental activity, sensory distortions, hallucinations, jaw tension, sweating.

**Tolerance and Dependence:** physical dependence to MDA is not likely because of the tolerance factor. This would leave MDA chronic abuse to a moderate psychological dependence, although this can vary. The variable factors include on the individuals specific reactions, the potency of the drug, and why it is being used.

Tolerance to MDA, as with the other hallucinogens, is high. For this reason, chronic use or abuse of MDA is not prevalent, but may be at a higher risk if it is used in moderate doses in which it will act as a stimulant, rather than an hallucinogen.

## MDE or MDEA (N-monoethyl-methylenedioxyamphetamine) - by users, this drug has been named Eve. When taken, an initial rush is followed by increased activity, which can result in muscle spasms. This is then followed by the actual high. The use of this drug has proven a greater risk of miscarriages.

## MDMA (methylenedioxymethamphetamine) - is a synthetic drug related to amphetamine and the hallucinogens.

In the 1970's and early 1980's psychiatrists employed it to facilitate psychotherapy, but soon after it was found to be toxic to the nervous systems of laboratory animals and was banned from medical use by the Food and Drug Administration.

The most common name used to refer to this drug is "ecstasy." Other names by which it is known are XTC, Adam, E, or EA-1475; which is the name given to it by the U.S. Army.

When it is taken (as a yellow tablet), the following effects may occur: extreme restlessness and agitation, fatigue, convulsions, a feeling of closeness to others, the user may become more verbal and communication skills seem to be improved.

Also, MDMA causes a less restful and less total sleep as compared to ones normal sleep schedule.

A few deaths have been reported as a result of overdose.

**TMA (3,4,5-trimethoxyamphetamine)** - is a synthetic mescaline analog. Its effects are similar to those of mescaline, but TMA is about 2 times more potent. TMA-2 is also similar, but is about 17 times more potent.

### Helpful Natural Treatments:

*Vitamins:* A, B complex, B3, B5, B12, C, Sodium ascorbate (buffered vitamin C) and E.

*Minerals:* Calcium, Magnesium (chelated form) and Selenium.

*Aminos:* L-Glutathione, L-Lithium carbonate & L-Phenylalanine.

*Foods:* dark green leaves, flax, hemp seed, pumpkin seed, soy bean and walnut.

*Herbs:* Astragalus, Cayenne, Cowslip, Echinacea, Ginseng, Hops, Licorice Root, Lobelia, Milk Thistle, Pau D'Arco, Siberian Ginseng, Golden Seal, Suma, Valerian Root, and Yucca.

*Also:* a high potency multivitamin; a high potency mineral complex; GABA (gamma-aminobutyric acid); Red Spearmint. This herb can help to safely alleviate restlessness associated with withdrawal symptoms.

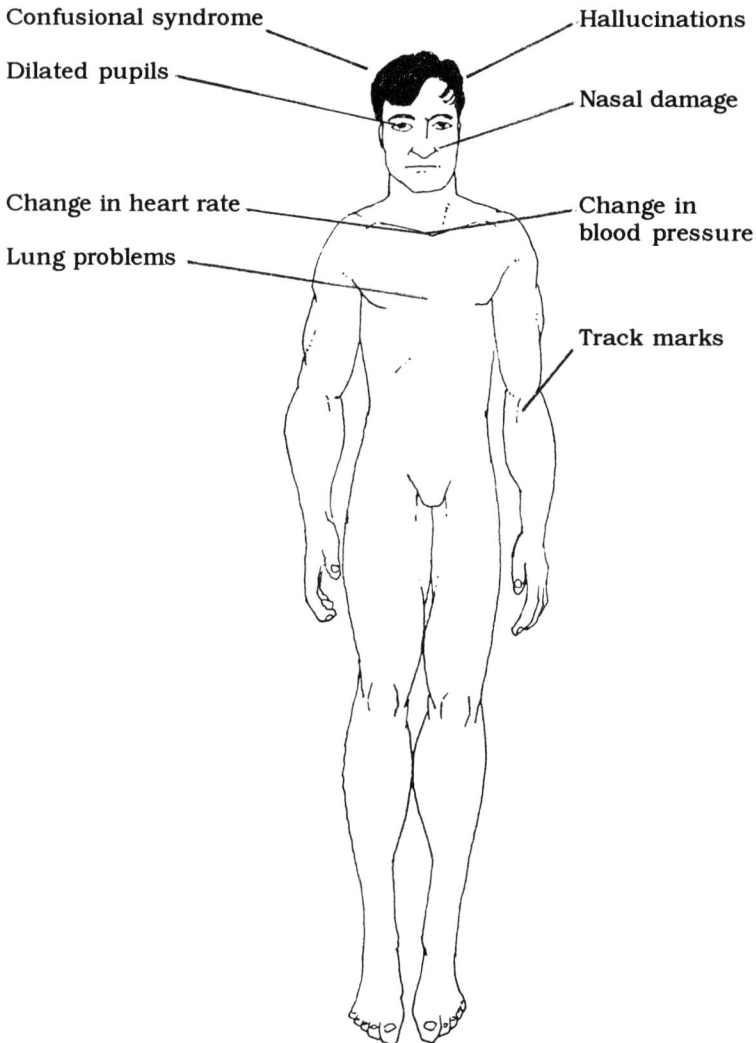

Confusional syndrome

Hallucinations

Dilated pupils

Nasal damage

Change in heart rate

Change in blood pressure

Lung problems

Track marks

Adverse effects and problem areas associated
with short and long term use of
**DMT/DET**
*Dimethyltryptamine - Diethytryptamine*

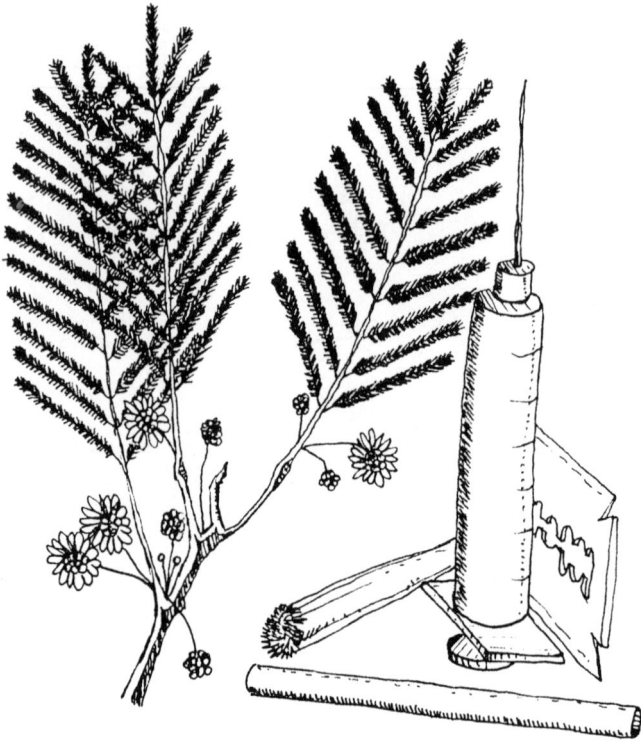

# OTHER HALLUCINOGENS

***Diethyltryptamine (DET) and Dimethyltryptamine (DMT)*** - these are both chemical analogs of tryptamine, a substance which has been found to exist in natural resources all over the world. DMT has been discovered to exist in nature whereas DET has not.

Dimethyltryptamine is structurally similar to psilocybin and is present in hallucinogenic drinks made from South American shrubs.

Because the effects last only a short while, it can be used during a lunch break and therefore has been given the name *businessman's trip* or *businessman's special.*

DMT is not absorbed through the skin and into the bloodstream when taken orally. For this reason, it is usually inhaled as a powder or as smoke from a cigarette, but can also be injected. Most commonly, it is soaked in parsley and dried prior to it being smoked.

It is an active ingredient in various South American snuffs, such as *yopo* and *cohoba*. The leaves and seeds are dried and powdered into a snuff that produce a short, intense hallucinatory experience.

**Derivatives:** diethyltryptamine, dimethyltryptamine.

**Brand Names:** dimethyltryptamine, diethyltryptamine.

**Street Names:** businessman's trip, businessman's special.

**Medical Advantages:** none.

**Illegal Applications:** the manufacturing, selling, purchasing, injecting, or inhaling these drugs.

**Appearance and Methods of Use:** smoking, snorting, or solution prepared for injection.

**Short Term Effects:** when using the psychedelic dose of 50 mg. or more, it takes from 5 to 20 minutes for the drug to take effect and the effects usually last from 10 to 30 minutes, depending on the method of use. Hallucinations and confusional syndrome which follow inhalation are due, partly, because of this drug, although bufotenine, which is also present, adds to the effects.

The effects produced by this drug are very similar to LSD, but last only about 10 minutes, when inhaled.

Another similar aspect to LSD is that the user may have a panic reaction, but because of the short duration of effects, this quickly wares off.

Other effects brought on by DMT are intense feelings, change in blood pressure, dilated pupils, sudden, more intense thoughts and visions.

**Long Term Effects:** possible lung problems due to inhalation, but if injected it may cause other problems as well.

**Tolerance and Dependence:** it is not known if tolerance is developed with DMT or DET use, but if there is, it is very gradual because of the short duration of effects. The user does not become physically dependent to DMT or DET, but mild psychological dependence may be developed.

# "Drugs and Beyond"

**Mappine (Bufotenine)** - is a derivative of tryptamine which can be found in significant amounts in many toad species and can be obtained from the secretion of these amphibians' skin.

It is also found, in small amounts, in the mushrooms Amanita muscaria and Amanita mappa, and in the seeds of the Piptadenia peregrina tree, which is found in Haiti and Venezuela. It is usually made into snuff in which the powder is blown into the nostrils through long tubes. Other methods are to make it into a solution for injection (which is taken intravenously) or added to various drinks which must be combined with MAO inhibitors (see clinical antidepressants) to be active orally.

Which ever way it is used, the effects are intense and very similar to LSD, but do not usually last as long.

### Helpful Natural Treatments:

*Vitamins:* A, B complex, B3, B5, B12, C, Sodium ascorbate (buffered vitamin C) and E.

*Minerals:* Calcium, Magnesium (chelated form) and Selenium.

*Aminos:* L-Glutathione, L-Lithium carbonate & L-Phenylalanine.

*Foods:* dark green leaves, flax, hemp seed, pumpkin seed, soy bean and walnut.

*Herbs:* Astragalus, Cayenne, Cowslip, Echinacea, Ginseng, Hops, Licorice Root, Lobelia, Milk Thistle, Pau D'Arco, Siberian Ginseng, Golden Seal, Suma, Valerian Root, and Yucca.

*Also:* a high potency multivitamin; a high potency mineral complex; GABA (gamma-aminobutyric acid); Red Spearmint. This herb can help to safely alleviate restlessness associated with withdrawal symptoms.

Brain damage

Emotional Instability

Central nervous system damage

Development of cancers

Pancreatic disorders

Increased urine output

Liver damage

Hangover

Drowsiness

Incoherent speech

Heart disease

Nausea & vomiting

Development of ulcers

Birth defects

Staggered walk

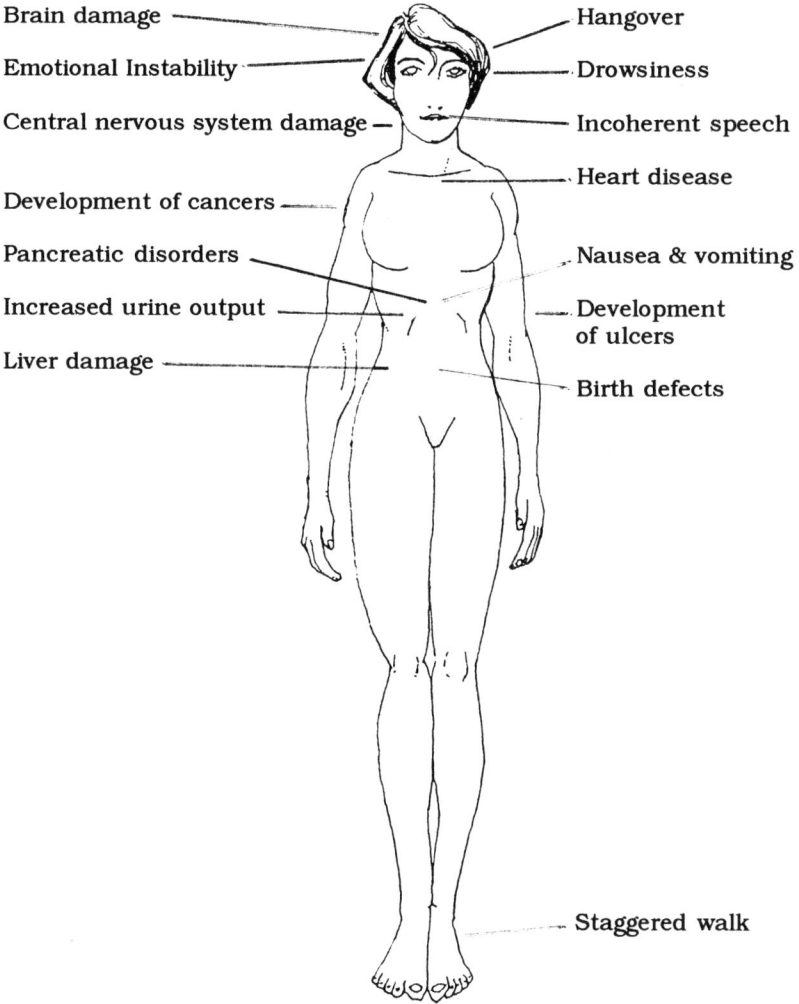

Adverse effects and problem areas associated
with short and long term use of
*Alcohol*

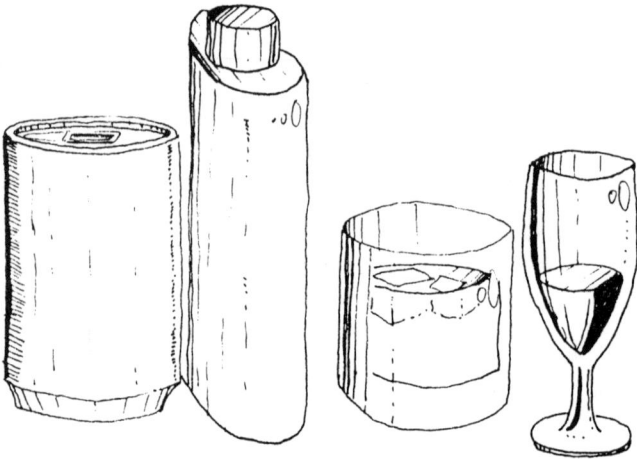

# CENTRAL NERVOUS SYSTEM (CNS) DEPRESSANTS AND SEDATIVE-HYPNOTIC COMPOUNDS

***ALCOHOL*** - is a colorless liquid produced from the fermentation of carbohydrates by yeast. Also known as ethanol or ethyl alcohol, it is the active constituent of alcoholic drinks such as beer, wine and hard liquors (spirits).

In medicine, alcohol is used as an antiseptic and a solvent.

***Note:*** many over-the-counter medications for colds contain alcohol. The alcohol in these medicines does deplete important vitamins and minerals. See Helpful Natural Treatments for depleted vitamins and minerals.

***Derivatives:*** ethyl alcohol or ethanol.

***Brand Names:*** all commercial hard liquors (spirits), wines and malts.

**Street Names:** booze, shot, two-six, forty, forty pounder, sixty, sixty pounder and many other names used to describe drinks concocted of different alcohols.

**Medical Advantages:** increases metabolic rate, thins blood, sedates, promotes sleep and is a good food source of energy.

**Illegal Applications:** purchasing alcoholic beverages which are contraband or home brewed or selling these for profit; driving or operating machinery while intoxicated; selling alcoholic beverages to minors.

**Appearance And Methods Of Use:** drank as a beverage and can appear in many different colors.

**Behavioral Characteristics:** usually lives the night life (they spend most of their time drinking at night), loss of personal possessions (sold to buy alcohol), drop in grades, increased illness (actually, the person is not usually sick, as such, but may have a hangover), unusual borrowing of money, mood swings, change of friends, loss of interest in former goals, difficulty in concentrating, slurred speech and possible personality change. Possible use of visine to clear the redness of the eyes and the use of chewing gum or candy which will have a strong odor-killing scent so the smell of alcohol cannot be detected. Also see "Short Term and Long Term Effects" for further evidence of abuse.

**Short Term Effects:** effects the brain and spinal cord in proportion to the amount of alcohol in the bloodstream. Euphoria, drowsiness, dizziness, slurred speech, staggering, stupor, headache, nausea, shakiness and vomiting. Alcohol should not be taken with any other drugs as physical and/or mental damage may occur; i.e. - if alcohol is taken with aspirin, it may increase the internal bleeding.

**Long Term Effects:** liver damage, brain damage, heart disease, certain types of cancer, loss of memory, impotence, ulcers and pancreatic disorders.
   Alcohol can irritate the mucous lining in a persons stomach and produce gastritis (symptoms being loss of appetite, nausea, vomiting and discomfort after eating) which will usually go away after the cause has been removed.

# "Drugs and Beyond"

**Note:** If the users symptoms persist to the extreme: empty stomach contents, maintain body heat, give the person hot black coffee, perform artificial respiration (mouth-to-mouth respiration) and any other support needed and seek medical help.

Symptoms of overdose include extreme disorientation and stupor, inability to speak coherently, inability to walk, loss of bladder and bowel control, severe weakness, life-threatening cardiovascular and respiratory depression, coma and possibly death if not treated immediately.

See "**Note**" above if overdose is suspected and seek medical help immediately.

**NOTE:** *Fetal Alcohol Syndrome* is a disorder in which a proportion of alcohol a mother drinks is reached by the unborn child and increases the chances of the child's abnormal development within the womb.

An affected baby is abnormally short, has small eyes and jaw and may have heart defects, a cleft lip and palate and lower-than-normal intelligence. The baby may suck poorly, sleep badly and be irritable.

The damage that alcohol can cause has only recently been recognized. Drinking more than 2 alcoholic drinks a day will increase the chance of a child being affected with the disorder, especially in the early months. This level of drinking may also cause a miscarriage; occasional drinking may cause the same effects.

Also, a link between alcohol and breast cancer has been recognized. Estrogen is a powerful hormone that promotes cellular growth in breast and reproductive tissue. It is believed that continual exposure of estrogen and breast tissue may be the root of the problem. Premenopausal women who have 2 or more drinks a day have higher levels of estrogen in their urine. This means that the risk of contracting breast cancer may be increased.

**Tolerance and Dependence:** chronic misuse of alcohol lowers mood and often leads to suicidal tendencies in the user. Yet this is often overlooked by doctors approached by people showing signs of depression. One should be cautious and carefully observe anyone possessing these signs.

Note: for symptoms of depression, see antidepressants.

The dependence of alcohol can be divided into 4 phases.
In the first phase, tolerance develops in the heavy social drinker.

The second phase consists of the drinker experiencing memory lapses relating to events occurring during the drinking episodes, also known as blackouts.

In the third phase, there is a lack or loss of control over alcohol. The drinker can no longer be certain of discontinuing drinking whenever he or she wants to.

The fourth and final phase is characterized by prolonged binges of intoxication and by observable mental or physical complications.

Alcohol withdrawal can have severe symptoms, but the severity of the symptoms is different from person to person depending on ones dependency to alcohol. Symptoms may include rapid heart rate, shortness of breath, chills, fever of 100.5 degrees Fahrenheit, chest pain, nausea with recurrent vomiting, abdominal pain, hallucinations and seizures. The bodies reaction to withdrawal can be divided into 4 stages.

The first stage usually sets in from 6 to 12 hours after the last drink. Anxiety, restlessness, sweating, increased heart rate, difficulty sleeping and increased blood pressure are common. Dependency is not extreme at this point and discomforts may be minor and treatable without medication; reassurance may be extremely beneficial.

In stage 2, the symptoms begin after 12 hours and peak at 24 to 36 hours. The symptoms include those from stage 1 along with visual and auditory hallucinations, notable because of relatively clear intervals. When not hallucinating, the person is well oriented and aware of having hallucinated. Medical treatment should always be sought at this stage.

In stage 3, which begins 12 to 48 hours after the last drink, seizures may occur. In some individuals, these may appear as early as 7 hours after the last drink.

In 72 to 96 hours after the last drink (stage 4), delirium and tremors (delirium tremens or DT's) appear, which consists of increasing confusion, disorientation, agitation and paranoid hallucinations.

Treatment must be sought or the DT's may persist for several days and death may occur in as much as 50% of the time, especially when there is an underlying medical problem. Recovery usually takes 5 to 7 days. A person with an alcohol-dependent problem will, usually, not admit to it, try to do it on their own and, since they will not seek medical help, may cause severe damage to themselves. This is why family and friends should be alert to withdrawal symptoms of the alcohol-dependent person.

If these symptoms listed above are detected, medical help is **necessary**. This can be achieved by contacting your local doctor or group programs such as Alcoholics Anonymous which will give support to the user and the family and ease the user off of this drug.

There are also drugs that are in the experimental stages which could be extremely beneficial in helping the user get off of the alcohol addiction, i.e. - Naltrexone - a drug also used for Heroin addiction.

**Note:** alcohol should not be taken with any medication, drug or other substance which depresses the body. This has the potential for overdose and may cause death. See *Long-Term Effects* for help if an overdose occurs. Also, alcohol should not be taken with any strong stimulant for this could, if both are taken in large amounts, counteract each other leading to severe damage to the body, possibly even death.

### Helpful Natural Treatments:

*Vitamins:* A, B complex, B1, B2, B3, B5, B6, B9, B12, Choline, C, Pangamic acid, Sodium ascorbate (buffered vitamin C), D, E and K.

*Minerals:* Calcium, Chromium, Iron, Magnesium (chelated form), Manganese, Selenium and Zinc.

*Aminos:* L-Glutathione, L-Lithium carbonate & L-Phenylalanine.

*Foods:* dark green leaves, flax, hemp seed, pumpkin seed, soy bean and walnut.

*Herbs:* Astragalus, Cayenne, Cowslip, Echinacea, Ginseng, Hops, Licorice Root, Lobelia, Milk Thistle, Pau D'Arco, Siberian Ginseng, Golden Seal, Suma, Valerian Root, and Yucca.

*Also:* a high potency multivitamin; a high potency mineral complex; GABA (gamma-aminobutyric acid); Red Spearmint. This herb can help to safely alleviate restlessness associated with withdrawal symptoms.

Brain damage

Drowsiness

Blurred vision

Dry mouth

Perspiration

Nausea and/or vomiting

Birth complications

Emotional instability

Hallucinations & paranoia

Incoherent speech

Irregular heart rhythms

Diarrhea & constipation

Shuffled walk

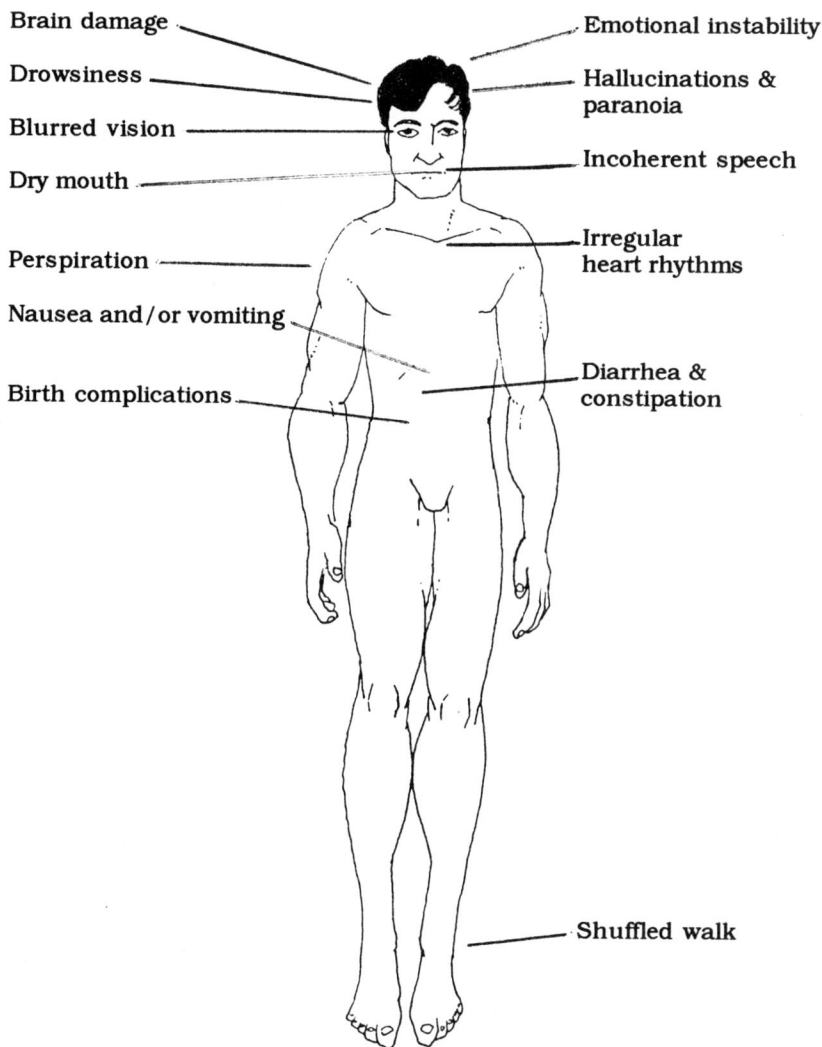

Adverse effects and problem areas associated
with short and long term use of
*Barbiturates*

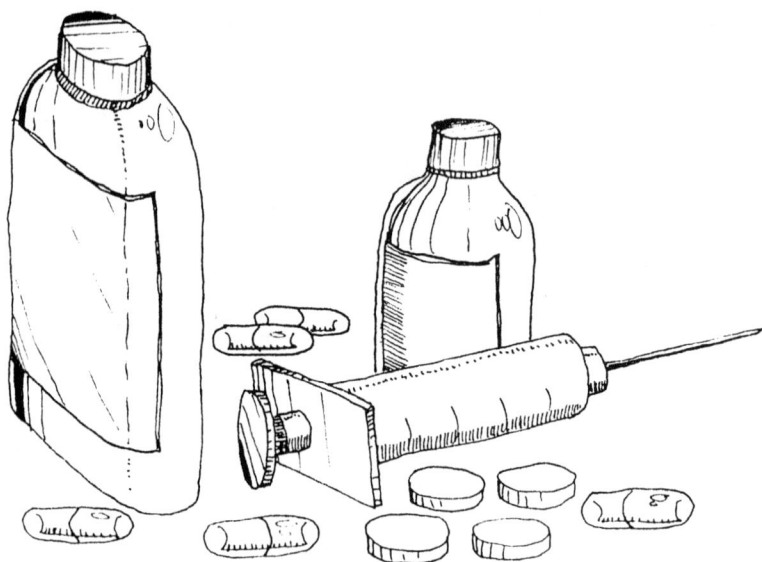

# BARBITURATES

**BARBITURATES** - a class of drugs that act as sedatives or induce sleep. These drugs depress the respiratory rate, blood pressure, temperature and nervous system. Hangovers have often been reported after barbiturate-induced sleep.

*Derivatives:* Amobarbital, Aprobarbital, Butabarbital (Butisol Sodium), Mephobarbital, Metharbital, Pentobarbital, Phenobarbital, Secobarbital and Secobarbital & Amobarbital.

*Brand Name: Amobarbital* (Amytal), *Aprobarbital* (Alurate), *Butabarbital* (Butalan, Butisol, Sarisol No. 2), *Mephobarbital* (Mebaral), *Metharbital* (Gemonil), *Pentobarbital* (Nembutal, Nova Rectal, Novopentobarb), *Phenobarbital* (Ancalixir, Barbita, Luminal, Solfoton), *Secobarbital* (Novosecobarb, Seconal), *Secobarbital* and *Amobarbital* (Tuinal).

*Street Names:* Barbs, biscuits, block busters, blue birds, blue devils, blue heaven, blues (Amytal), bullets, christmas trees, dolls, downers, downs, fool pills, goof balls, goofers, green dragons, greenies, Mexican reds, nemmies, pajao, phennies, pink ladies, purple hearts, rainbows, red birds, red devils, reds (Seconal), rojo, seccies, shorties, sleepers, sleeping pills, stumblers, tooies, toolies, trees, tuiys, yellow jackets (Nembutal), yellows.

**Medical Advantages:** acute emotional distress, anxiety, depression, insomnia, muscle spasms, psychic disorders, to control chemically induced convulsions, tension, and daytime sedation. Some may be used before surgery to relieve anxiety and tension and others as anticonvulsants to help control seizures in certain disorders or diseases, such as epilepsy.

**Illegal Applications:** sold, purchased, prescribed, or consumed without authorization from proper authorities.

**Appearance And Methods Of Use:** barbiturates are usually taken orally in capsule, elixir or tablet forms, but can be taken by injection or as a suppository.

**Behavioral Characteristics:** perspiration, drop in grades, mood swings, increased illness, dizziness, irritability, unusual borrowing of money, sloppy dress, loss of personal possessions (sold to buy drugs), hallucinations, drowsiness, weight gain, loss of interest in former goals, confusion, slurred speech, difficulty in concentrating, nausea and vomiting, and change of friends. Also see "Short Term and Long Term Effects" for further evidence of abuse.

**Short Term Effects:** drowsiness, dizziness, confusion, nausea, diarrhea or constipation, dry mouth, palpitations, elevated or lowered blood sugar levels, hallucinations, sweating, nightmares, urine retention, weight gain, blurred vision, slurred speech, irregular heart rhythms and irritability.

**Long Term Effects:** common chronic symptoms that may develop with prolonged use are shortened memory, constant drowsiness, loss of coordination and awareness, emotional instability, slurred speech, paranoia, coma, brain damage and possibly death.

**Tolerance and Dependence:** tolerance develops when the drug is taken in repeated short intervals. Physical dependence is prevalent when the drug is taken in above recommended levels for 1 to 2 months or longer. Psychological dependence also exists because of their minimal side effects.

# "Drugs and Beyond"

Barbiturates are very addicting and create severe withdrawal symptoms. Anxiety is usually the first symptom, followed by the person becoming increasingly violent and, depending on how dependent the user has become, can result in seizures and even death. Other symptoms include: restlessness, nausea and vomiting, insomnia, delusions and convulsions, abdominal cramps, shaking, delirium and weakness. Withdrawal should not be done personally; medical help must be sought.

Overdose is probable and symptoms include: a drastic drop in number of breaths taken per minute and a drastic drop in blood pressure, unconsciousness, coma and death. Medical help must be sought immediately when these symptoms are discovered.

**Note:** emptying stomach contents, artificial respiration or mouth-to-mouth resuscitation, maintaining body heat and any other support which can be given to the victim will help to reverse these symptoms. Medical help must be sought immediately thereafter.

**Note:** never take barbiturates with alcohol. Even a small amount of barbiturates taken with alcohol can result in an overdose.

### Helpful Natural Treatments:

*Vitamins:* A, B, B complex, B1, B2, B3, B5, B6, B9, B12, Choline, C, Pangamic acid, Sodium ascorbate (buffered vitamin C), D, E and K.

*Minerals:* Calcium, Chromium, Iron, Magnesium (chelated form), Manganese, Selenium and Zinc.

*Aminos:* L-Glutathione, L-Lithium carbonate & L-Phenylalanine.

*Foods:* dark green leaves, flax, hemp seed, pumpkin seed, soy bean and walnut.

*Herbs:* Astragalus, Cayenne, Cowslip, Echinacea, Ginseng, Hops, Licorice Root, Lobelia, Milk Thistle, Pau D'Arco, Siberian Ginseng, Golden Seal, Suma, Valerian Root, and Yucca.

*Also:* a high potency multivitamin; a high potency mineral complex; GABA (gamma-aminobutyric acid); Red Spearmint. This herb can help to safely alleviate restlessness associated with withdrawal symptoms.

Light headedness

Blurred vision

Dry mouth

Emotional instability

Slurred speech

Rapid & weak pulse

Clumsiness

Trembling

Urination problems

Unsteadiness

Nausea or vomiting

Constipation
or diarrhea

Birth complications

Staggered walk

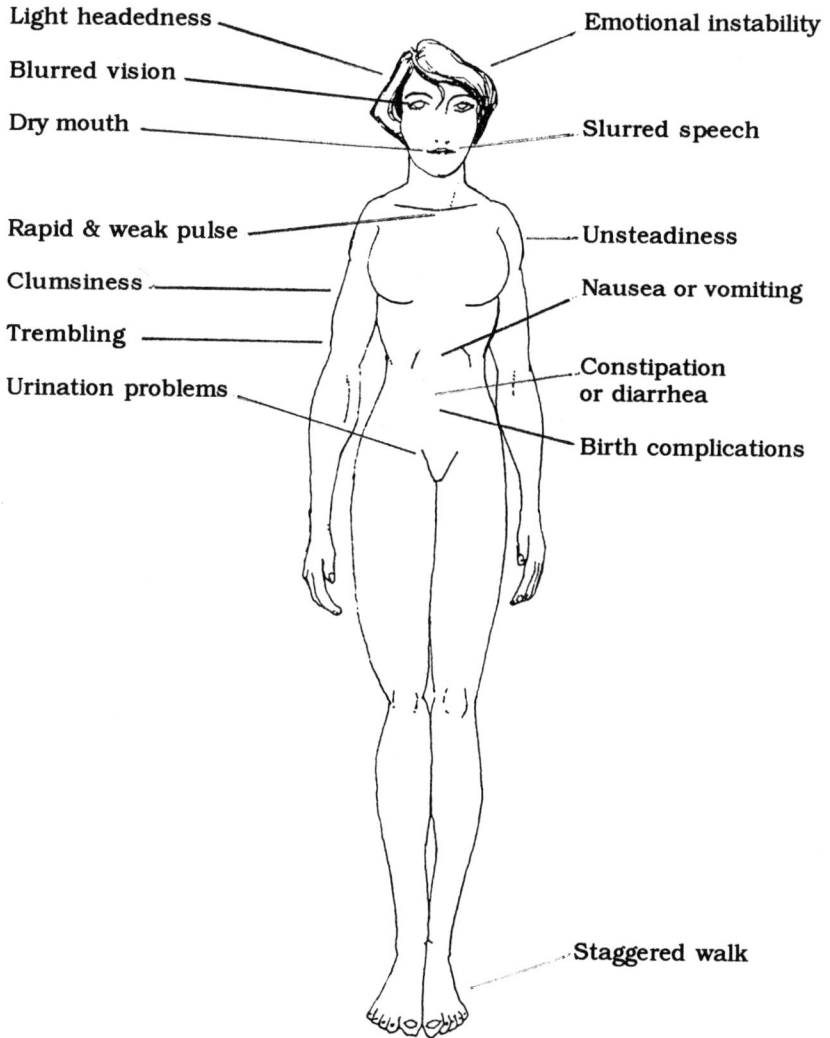

Adverse effects and problem areas associated
with short and long term use of
**Benzodiazepines / tranquilizers**

# "Drugs and Beyond"

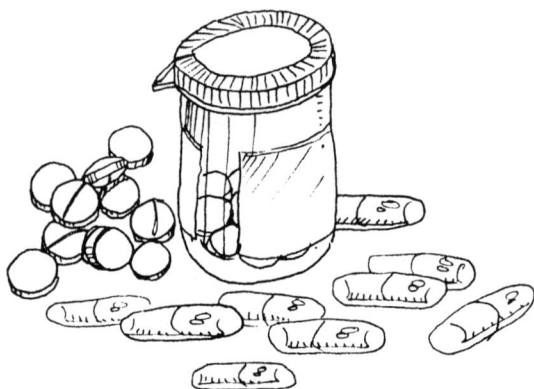

# BENZODIAZEPINES AND TRANQUILIZERS (NONBARBITURATE HYPNOTICS AND SEDATIVES)

**BENZODIAZEPINES** - are medicines which slow down the central nervous system.

**TRANQUILIZERS** - drugs which bring tranquillity by calming, soothing, quieting, or pacifying without depression.

***Derivatives:*** Alprazolam, Chlordiazepoxide, Chlorzoxazone and Acetaminophen, Clorazepate, Cyclobenzaprine, Diazepam, Flurazepam, Glutethimide, Meprobamate, Oxazepam, Prazepam, Temazepam, Triazolam.

***Brand Names: Alprazolam*** (Apo-Alpraz, Novo-Alprazol, Nu-Alpraz, Xanax); ***Chlordiazepoxide*** (Apo-Chlordiazepoxide, Libritabs, Librium, Lipoxide, Novopoxide, Solium); ***Chlorzoxazone*** and ***Acetaminophen*** (Chlorozoxozone with APAP, Parafon Forte); ***Clorazepate*** (Apo-Clorazepate, Gen-XENE, Novoclopate, Tranxene,

Tranxene-SD, Tranxene T-Tab); *Cyclobenzaprine* (Cycoflex, Flexeril); *Diazepam* (Apo-Diazepam, Diazemuls, Diazepam Intensol, Novodipam, PMS Diazepam, T-Quil, Valium, Valrelease, Vazepam, Vivol, Zetran); *Flurazepam* (Apo-Flurazepam, Dalmane, Durapam, Novoflupam, Somnol); *Glutethimide* (Dorigulate); *Meprobamate* (Acabamate, Apo-Meprobamate, Equanil, Meditran, Meprospan 200, Meprospan 400, Meprospan-400, Miltown, 'Miltown'-200, 'Miltown'-400, 'Miltown'-600, Neuramate, Novomepro, Probate, Sedabamate, Trancot); *Oxazepam* (Apo-Oxazepam, Novoxapam, Serax, Zapex); *Prazepam* (Centrax); *Temazepam* (Razepam, Restoril); *Triazolam* (Apo-Triazo, Halcion, Novotriolam, Nu-Triazo).

**Street Names:** unknown.

**Medical Advantages:** some are used to relieve nervousness or tension, but not if the nervousness and tension are due to stress of every day life. Others are used in the treatment of insomnia and to treat certain convulsive disorders, like epilepsy; although, for insomnia, they are usually only effective for a few weeks.

Alprazolam is used in the treatment of panic disorder and diazepam is used to relax tense muscles and to relieve muscle spasm.

Benzodiazepines may also be used for other conditions which would be determined by a doctor.

**Illegal Applications:** selling, purchasing, or consuming benzodiazepines without authorization from proper authorities.

**Appearance And Methods Of Use:** this type of drug can be taken: orally by tablet (sublingual or otherwise), capsule (extended release or otherwise), or oral solution; by injection; or by rectal solution.

**Behavioral Characteristics:** difficulty in concentrating, clumsiness, drop in grades, mood swings, lightheadedness, increased illness, unusual borrowing of money, weight loss, dizziness, slurred speech, loss of interest in former goals, sloppy dress, unsteadiness, loss of personal possessions (sold to buy drugs) and a change of friends. Also see "Short Term and Long Term Effects" for further evidence of abuse.

**Short Term Effects:** abdominal cramps, increased bronchial secretions, lightheadedness, urination problems, blurred vision, clumsiness, slurred speech, trembling, headache, dry mouth, nausea or vomiting, pounding or fast heartbeat, unusual weakness or tiredness, loss or change in sexual desire, constipation, muscle spasms, dizziness, diarrhea, drowsiness, a sense of well-being.

**Long Term Effects:** slurred speech, emotional instability, constant drowsiness, shortened memory, loss of coordination and awareness and paranoia.

**Tolerance And Dependence:** when benzodiazepines have been used for a prolonged period of time, they can produce physical dependence, psychological dependence, and tolerance quite rapidly, creating withdrawal symptoms similar to those of barbiturates, but less severe. This will vary depending on the dosage, the specific drug used, and duration of use.

### Helpful Natural Treatments:

*Vitamins:* A, B complex, B1, B2, B3, B5, B6, B9, B12, Choline, C, Pangamic acid, Sodium ascorbate (buffered vitamin C), D, E and K.

*Minerals:* Calcium, Chromium, Iron, Magnesium (chelated form), Manganese, Selenium and Zinc.

*Aminos:* L-Glutathione, L-Lithium carbonate & L-Phenylalanine.

*Foods:* dark green leaves, flax, hemp seed, pumpkin seed, soy bean and walnut.

*Herbs:* Astragalus, Cayenne, Cowslip, Echinacea, Ginseng, Hops, Licorice Root, Lobelia, Milk Thistle, Pau D'Arco, Siberian Ginseng, Golden Seal, Suma, Valerian Root, and Yucca.

*Also:* a high potency multivitamin; a high potency mineral complex; GABA (gamma-aminobutyric acid); Red Spearmint. This herb can help to safely alleviate restlessness associated with withdrawal symptoms.

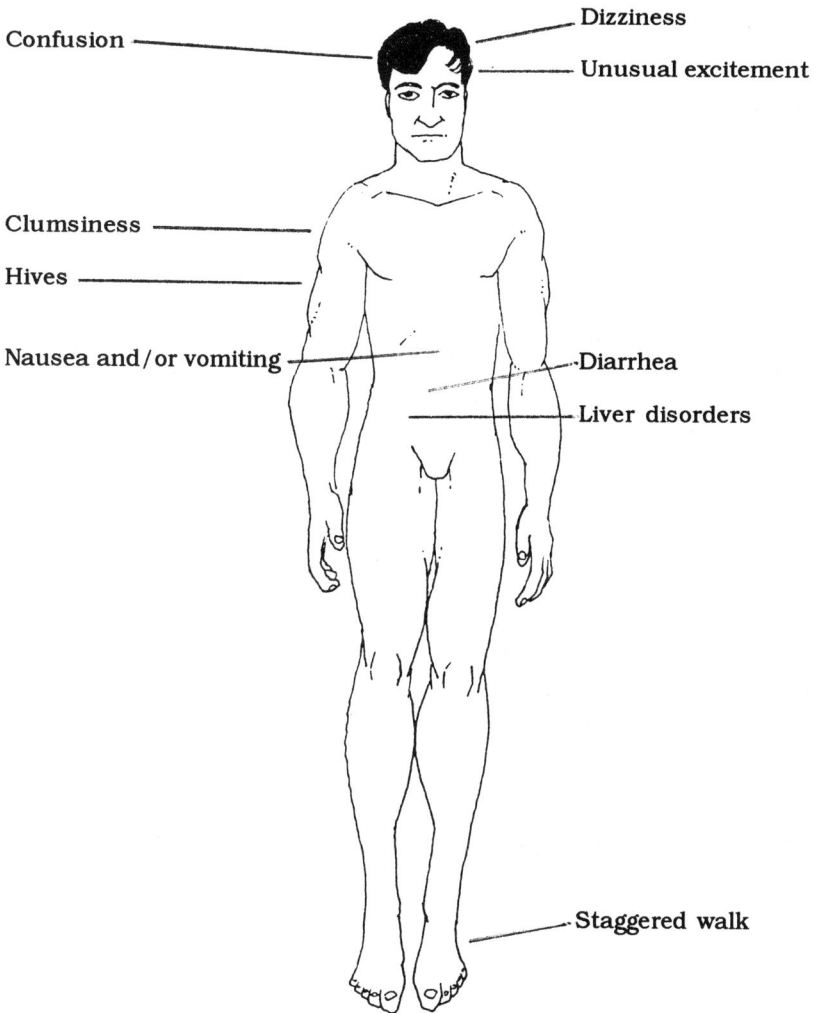

Confusion

Dizziness

Unusual excitement

Clumsiness

Hives

Nausea and/or vomiting

Diarrhea

Liver disorders

Staggered walk

Adverse effects and problem areas associated
with short and long term use of
*Chloral Hydrate*

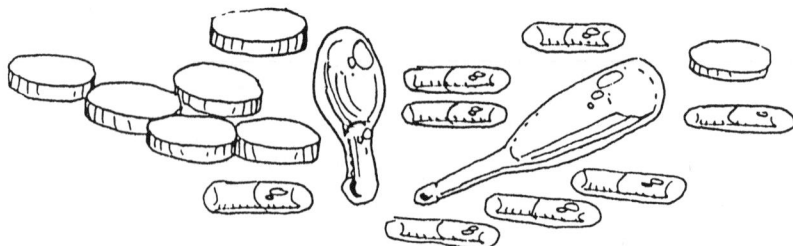

# CHLORAL HYDRATE

**Chloral Hydrate -** is a sedative-hypnotic compound which was first synthesized in 1832 and is sometimes used before surgery to help relieve anxiety and tension, in the treatment of insomnia, and has been used in the treatment of alcohol withdrawal. It is not used very often in medicine since it has been replaced by other medicines used to treat these problems.

***Derivatives:*** chloral hydrate.

***Brand Names:*** Aquachloral Supprettes, Noctec, Novochlorhydrate.

***Street Names:*** green frogs, knockout drops, peter.

***Medical Advantages:*** used in the treatment of anxiety and tension in presurgery and in the treatment of insomnia.

***Illegal Applications:*** consuming, administering, selling or purchasing chloral hydrate without authorization from proper authorities.

***Appearance and Methods of Use:*** can be taken orally as capsules or syrup or in suppository form.

***Behavioral Characteristics:*** irritability, drop in grades, sloppy dress, unusual borrowing of money, mood swings, difficulty in concentrating, constant cough, increased illness, change of friends, loss of personal possessions (sold to buy drugs), weight loss, loss of interest in former goals and slurred speech. Also see "Short Term and Long Term Effects" for further evidence of abuse.

**Short Term Effects:** clumsiness, confusion, diarrhea, dizziness, grogginess, hallucinations, hives, lightheadedness, nausea and vomiting, skin rash, stomach pain, and unusual excitement.

**Long Term Effects:** liver problems with extended use and death from an overdose.

**Tolerance and Dependence:** some physical and psychological dependence is developed through the use of chloral hydrate and moderate tolerance is developed over time.

### Helpful Natural Treatments:

*Vitamins:* A, B, B complex, B1, B2, B3, B5, B6, B9, B12, Choline, C, Pangamic acid, Sodium ascorbate (buffered vitamin C), D, E and K.

*Minerals:* Calcium, Chromium, Iron, Magnesium (chelated form), Manganese, Selenium and Zinc.

*Aminos:* L-Glutathione, L-Lithium carbonate & L-Phenylalanine.

*Foods:* dark green leaves, flax, hemp seed, pumpkin seed, soy bean and walnut.

*Herbs:* Astragalus, Cayenne, Cowslip, Echinacea, Ginseng, Hops, Licorice Root, Lobelia, Milk Thistle, Pau D'Arco, Siberian Ginseng, Golden Seal, Suma, Valerian Root, and Yucca.

*Also:* a high potency multivitamin; a high potency mineral complex; GABA (gamma-aminobutyric acid); Red Spearmint. This herb can help to safely alleviate restlessness associated with withdrawal symptoms.

## "Drugs and Beyond"

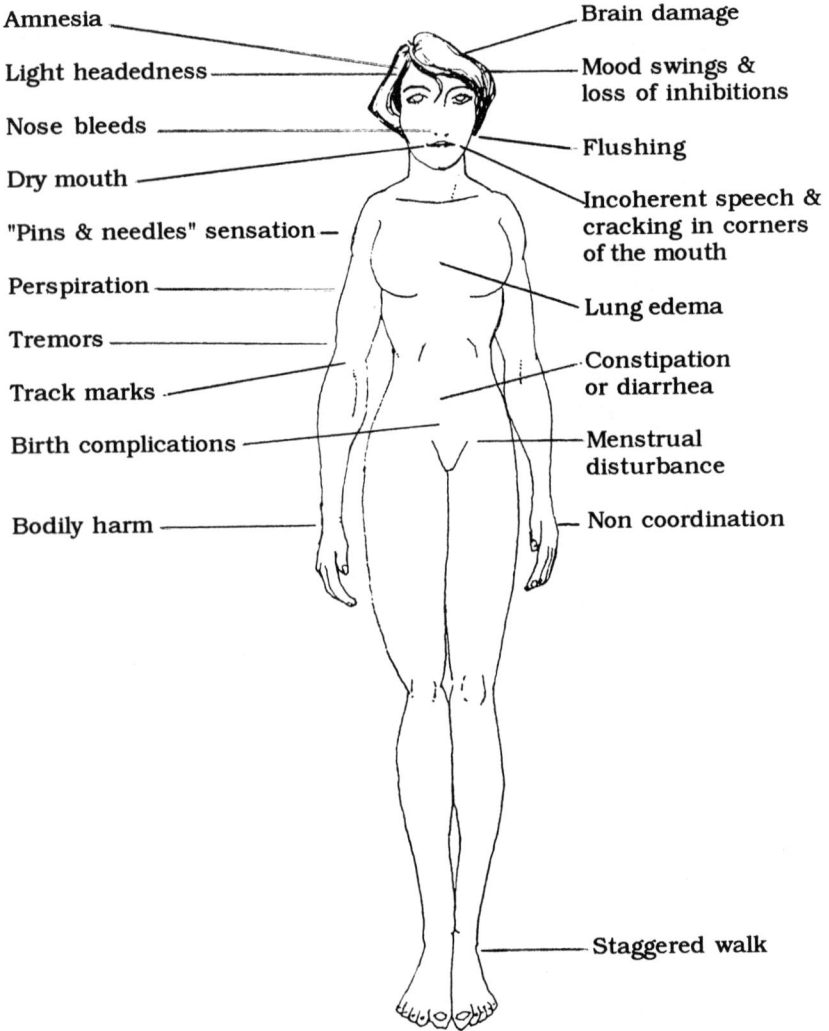

Amnesia

Light headedness

Nose bleeds

Dry mouth

"Pins & needles" sensation

Perspiration

Tremors

Track marks

Birth complications

Bodily harm

Brain damage

Mood swings & loss of inhibitions

Flushing

Incoherent speech & cracking in corners of the mouth

Lung edema

Constipation or diarrhea

Menstrual disturbance

Non coordination

Staggered walk

Adverse effects and problem areas associated with short and long term use of
### Methaqualone

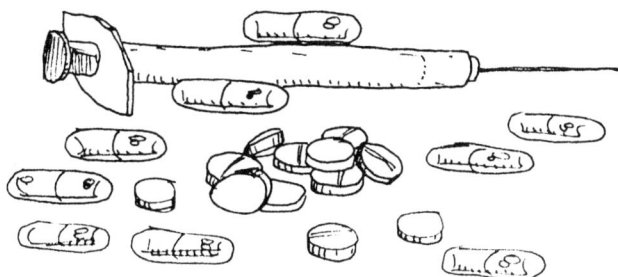

# METHAQUALONE

**METHAQUALONE (*Quaaludes*)** - methaqalone is 2-methyl-3-o-tolyl-4 (3H)-quinazoline. Quaaludes or methaqualone are non-barbiturate sedative-hypnotics. They act on a different central nervous system site than other sleeping pills, such as barbiturates.

The body distributes them in fat, brain tissue and the liver; by reducing neural transmissions to the brain. They suppress REM (rapid eye movement) during dreams, causing deep sleep, though not necessarily restful. Quaaludes are fast-acting, but the users of this drug fight the drowsiness that occurs within 10 to 20 minutes, seeking the body - relaxing effects. Some effects include being relaxed to the point of noncoordination and not being able to speak without slurring words.

Though labeled as having aphrodisiacal qualities, quaaludes are actually an *anaphrodisiac*, which simply means opposite to the latter.

Addiction is possible within 2 weeks at a daily dosage of 300-600 mg. All it takes for an overdose is 8, 300 mg. tablets, but, although it is probable, this does not mean that it will result in death.

**Derivatives:** Methaqualone.

**Brand Name:** Mandrax, Melsedrin, Optimil, Parest, Quaalude, Somnafac, Sopor, Tuazolone.

**Street Names:** greens, ludes, mandrakes, mean, quacks, quads, quas, 714's, soapers, soaps.

# "Drugs and Beyond"

**Medical Advantages:** methaqualone has anticonvulsant, antispasmodic, local anesthetic, antihistaminic, anaphrodisiacal and antitussive properties and can be used for any combination of these ailments.

**Illegal Applications:** selling, purchasing, or consuming methaqualone without authorization from proper authorities.

**Appearance And Methods Of Use:** ingested in the form of pills or capsules, but can be taken intravenously.

**Behavioral Characteristics:** tremors, perspiration, loss of personal possessions (sold to buy drugs), drop in grades, dry mouth, sloppy dress, hangover, slurred speech, nausea and vomiting, mood swings, constant cough, headache, cracking at the corners of the mouth, increased illness, amnesia, change of friends, skin rash, unusual borrowing of money, loss of interest in former goals, dizziness, weight loss and difficulty in concentrating. Also see "Short Term and Long Term Effects" for further evidence of abuse.

**Short Term Effects:** inability to speak without slurring words, a state of relaxation to the point of noncoordination, amnesia, dry mouth, headache, dizziness, tremors, numbness or a "pins and needles" sensation, a dreamlike state coupled with the loss of personal identity, menstrual disturbance, hangover, urticarea, nosebleeds, diarrhea, vomiting, quiescence, relaxation, loss of inhibitions, loss of appetite, constipation, cracking at the corners of the mouth, nose bleeds, possible mild seizures, skin rash, itching, flushing and increased sweating. They are said to increase libido, prolong sexual excitement and lower sexual inhibitions. Methaqualone produces painless pleasant loss or failure of muscle coordination with feelings of indestructibility and euphoria. When quaaludes are taken with alcohol, the possibility of an overdose is great; symptoms include muscle spasms, delirium, extreme tension of the muscles or arteries, convulsions, tremors, stomach hemorrhage and possibly death.

**Long Term Effects:** lung edema which could lead to permanent damage to the lungs; brain damage; convulsions from overdose which may cause damage to the victim due to his/her head hitting a hard surface, getting a severe wound from swinging of the arms, legs or body and contacting a hard surface or item with extreme force, etc.; and coma from overdose which could lead to death.

**NOTE** - If an overdose is suspected (symptoms being convulsions, tremors and stomach hemorrhage), medical attention must be sought immediately; KEEP THE VICTIM AWAKE AT ALL COSTS!

**Tolerance and Dependence:** the methaqualone user develops tolerance to the sleep inducing effect quickly, especially if used nightly for sleep and may, over time, increase the dose to as much as 10 times the original amount. But if the user quits the drug or switches to another drug for a period of time, then returns to methaqualone, the bodies tolerance is lessened and what was once an average dose for the user, may now cause overdose, coma or even death.

Tolerance to the "high" or euphoric state sought by daytime users is developed quickly and the dosage must be increased along with frequency of ingestion to maintain the same pleasurable effects.

Individual sensitivity to methaqualone can vary considerably. Some users have died from taking 8 000 mg. while others have survived the effects of 22 000 mg.

Though the user must increase the amount of the drug needed to cause the same effect, the amount needed to cause death remains the same. This is especially true when the user combines the drug with alcohol or barbiturates. Since all depress the body which will eventually come to the point where the body cannot handle it and shuts down.

Psychological dependence can exist when irregular low dose intervals are taken or even when the drug is not taken at all. Physical dependence occurs when a large dose of methaqualone is taken over a period of time. When the use of the drug is suddenly stopped, withdrawal symptoms set in.

Withdrawal syndrome includes insomnia, abdominal cramps, anxiety, nightmares, headache, nausea, irritability and hallucinations. These symptoms usually only last for about 3 days unless the severity is much greater where the symptoms could last up to a week or more.

A person going through withdrawal must be treated under specialized conditions, for the risk of death is probable. The victim must be observed carefully and be administered nonbarbiturate sedative/hypnotics to control severe methaqualone withdrawal.

Because of the less undesirable effects of methaqualone, as compared to barbiturate and nonbarbiturate sedative/hypnotics, users of methaqualone preferred to use it over the other drugs and had difficulty in stopping the use of this drug.

# "Drugs and Beyond"

Other people hadn't discovered their dependence until use of the drug was depleted. Even after a long period of time, the individuals still needed or had very strong cravings for the drug. People who use the drug at a set dosage and do not change the dosage find themselves having great difficulty coping without the drug when it becomes scarce.

### Helpful Natural Treatments:

*Vitamins:* A, B complex, B1, B2, B3, B5, B6, B9, B12, Choline, C, Pangamic acid, Sodium ascorbate (buffered vitamin C), D, E and K.

*Minerals:* Calcium, Chromium, Iron, Magnesium (chelated form), Manganese, Selenium and Zinc.

*Aminos:* L-Glutathione, L-Lithium carbonate & L-Phenylalanine.

*Foods:* dark green leaves, flax, hemp seed, pumpkin seed, soy bean and walnut.

*Herbs:* Astragalus, Cayenne, Cowslip, Echinacea, Ginseng, Hops, Licorice Root, Lobelia, Milk Thistle, Pau D'Arco, Siberian Ginseng, Golden Seal, Suma, Valerian Root, and Yucca.

*Also:* a high potency multivitamin; a high potency mineral complex; GABA (gamma-aminobutyric acid); Red Spearmint. This herb can help to safely alleviate restlessness associated with withdrawal symptoms.

Destructive behavior & loss of inhibitions

Brain damage, emotional instability confusion, & hallucinations

Grogginess & blackouts

Nasal discharge & bleeding

Ringing of the ears

Heart disease & Lung disorders

Inflamed mucous membranes

Nerve damage

Fatigue, body rushes, tremors, & hot flashes

Nausea and/or vomiting

Bodily harm

Staggered walk

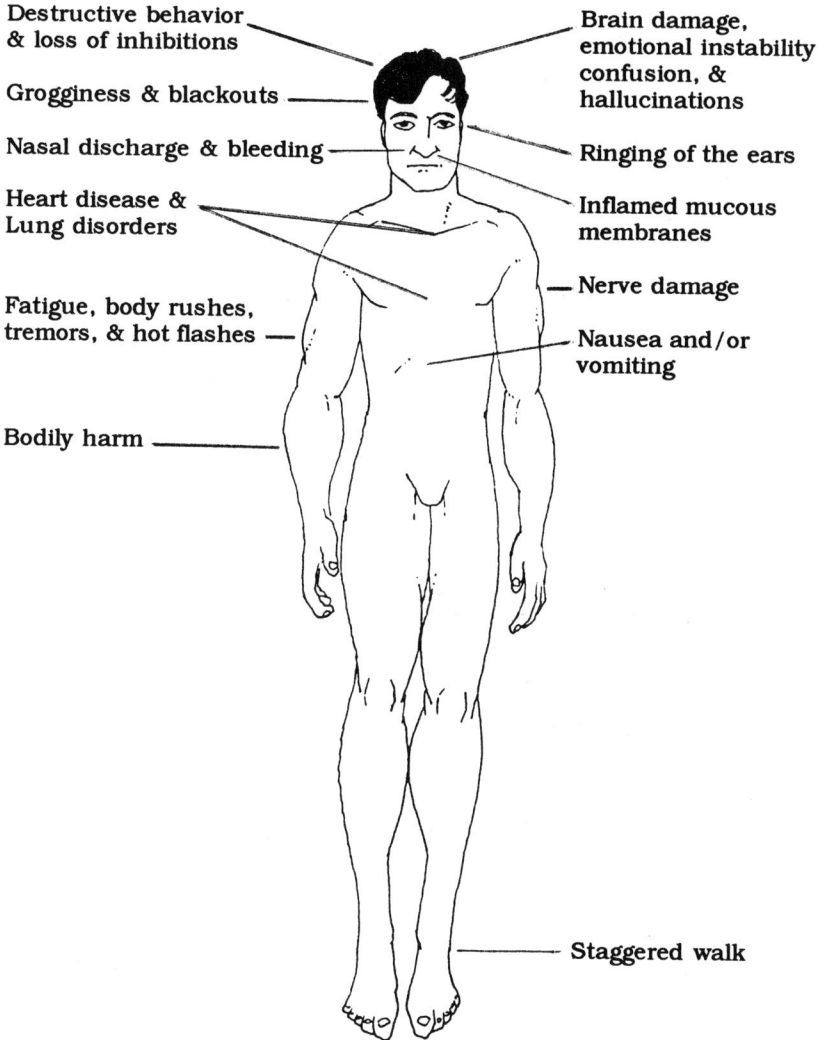

Adverse effects and problem areas associated with short and long term use of
## Volatile Inhalants

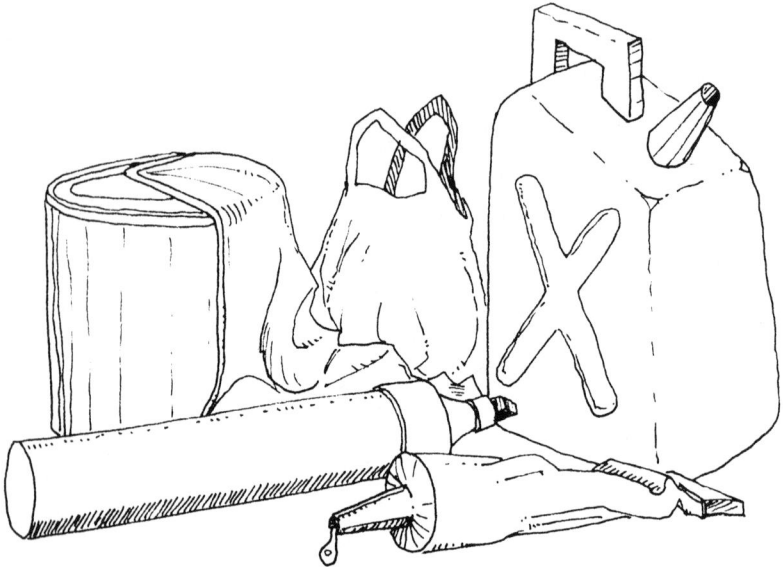

# VOLATILE INHALANTS
## (Deliriants)

**INHALANTS** - are solvent-based substances, such as glue, nail polish remover and gasoline, which can be sniffed to produce mind-altering effects. Though these substances are not classified as drugs, they are sometimes used as drugs and one should be cautious and be aware of their abuse potential.

Because children from the ages 7 to 17 are not legally allowed to drink alcohol or take certain drugs, they are the most common users of inhalants.

Users sniff solvents directly from the container; put solvent-soaked rags into a plastic bag, hold the bag to the mouth and inhale deeply or submerge their head completely into the bag. A person can suffocate and die if they become unconscious while the bag is still over their face or head.

**Derivatives:** Room deodorizers contain butyl and isobutyl nitrate (butyl nitrate is thought to intensify a sexual experience);

Amyl nitrate (a prescription drug, usually prescribed for the treatment of angina pectoris, which is a vasodilator that relaxes smooth muscle in small blood vessels, causing them to expand and so lower the blood pressure); freon (trichlorofluoromethane); nitrous oxide; halogenated hydrocarbons (i.e.., trichloroethylene); esters (i.e.., ethyl, amyl and butyl acetates); aromatic hydrocarbons (i.e.., benzene); volatile hydrocarbons of petroleum origin (i.e.. gasoline); acetone; chloroform; carbon tetrachloride; toluene; ether (ethyl oxide).

Nail polish remover; lighter fluids; cleaning fluids; airplane cement and any other volatile substance which, when inhaled, produce effects similar to the other commonly used inhalants.

**Brand Name:** all commercial products containing one or more chemicals listed in "derivatives" or any other volatile substance which can be inhaled to give the user a "high".

**Street Names:** ames, banapple gas, B-bombs, jac aroma, locker popper, locker room, pearls, poppers, rush, Satan's scent, snappers.

**Medical Advantages:** Nitrous oxide (laughing gas) is sometimes used to sedate a patient before an operation, but for the most part, these chemicals are too toxic and therefore too dangerous to be used for medicinal purposes.

Amyl nitrate is used to relieve pain from angina attacks.

**Illegal Applications:** any chemical substance sold with the know-ledge that it is going to be used to get the person high.

**Appearance And Methods Of Use:** inhaled from a plastic bag, a saturated cloth or directly.

**Behavioral Characteristics:** mood swings, increased amount of empty solvent container in the trash, disappearance of solvents from around the home, unusual borrowing of money, increased illness, loss of personal possessions (sold to buy inhalants), destructive behavior to self and to others, change of friends, signs of glue and other chemical stains on the face, hands, body and/or clothes, strong chemical smells on the breath of the user which may last for several hours after an episode,

# "Drugs and Beyond"

Weight loss, loss of interest in former goals, difficulty in concentrating, slurred speech, drop in grades, sloppy dress, accidents, lack of inhibition, sleepiness and an impaired recall of the drug induced events, generalized weakness and DEATH from cardiac arrhythmias, asphyxiation (suffocation because of lack of oxygen in the blood) and respiratory arrest. Also, see "Short Term and Long Term Effects for further evidence of abuse.

**Short Term Effects:** after a few seconds, the initial effects ware off, leaving the actual high lasting from 5 to 45 minutes. The effects include: dizziness, relaxation, mental confusion, lightheadedness, lack of coordination, fatigue, lack of inhibition, loss of appetite, blackouts, dysphoria, hallucinations, sleepiness, illusions, euphoria, nausea and well-being.

Slurred speech similar to alcohol is usually prevalent. There may also be hot flashes, body rushes, a feeling that one is floating and flashes of light.

People who inhale may become restless, uncoordinated and confused.

*Also:* laryngitis, tracheobronchitis, too little oxygen in the cells (hypoxia), cardiac irritability, inflamed sinuses, seizures, inflamed mucous membranes of the nose - with a nasal discharge, nosebleed, delirium, ringing of the ears, loss of muscle coordination, abdominal pain and visual impairment.

**Long Term Effects:** prolonged habitual use of inhalants can cause bloodshot eyes, nosebleeds, and the smell of chemicals on their breath. Personality changes and tremors can occur, as well as nerve damage, memory loss, heart disease, muscular weakness, hearing loss, fatigue, brain damage, development of cancerous tumors, vomiting and nausea. Also sudden death from inhalants has been reported.

**NOTE** - sucking inhalants directly from a tank or through a hose (i.e. - nitrous oxide or freon) can be disastrous because the rapidly expanding gas can easily freeze the lungs, cause the lungs to collapse or cause other serious damaging effects to the lungs.

**Tolerance and Dependence:** tolerance is built through the use of inhalants, but not to the damaging effects caused each time the solvent(s) are inhaled. The user may also become dependent on inhalants and will go through withdrawal symptoms which include hallucinations, chills and headaches.

Overdose from inhalants is prevalent and can be treated by artificial respiration or mouth-to-mouth respiration followed by immediate medical help.

### Helpful Natural Treatments:

*Vitamins:* A, B complex, B1, B2, B3, B5, B6, B9, B12, Choline, C, Pangamic acid, Sodium ascorbate (buffered vitamin C), D, E and K.

*Minerals:* Calcium, Chromium, Iron, Magnesium (chelated form), Manganese, Selenium and Zinc.

*Aminos:* L-Glutathione, L-Lithium carbonate & L-Phenylalanine.

*Foods:* dark green leaves, flax, hemp seed, pumpkin seed, soy bean and walnut.

*Herbs:* Astragalus, Cayenne, Cowslip, Echinacea, Ginseng, Hops, Licorice Root, Lobelia, Milk Thistle, Pau D'Arco, Siberian Ginseng, Golden Seal, Suma, Valerian Root, and Yucca.

*Also:* a high potency multivitamin; a high potency mineral complex; GABA (gamma-aminobutyric acid); Red Spearmint. This herb can help to safely alleviate restlessness associated with withdrawal symptoms.

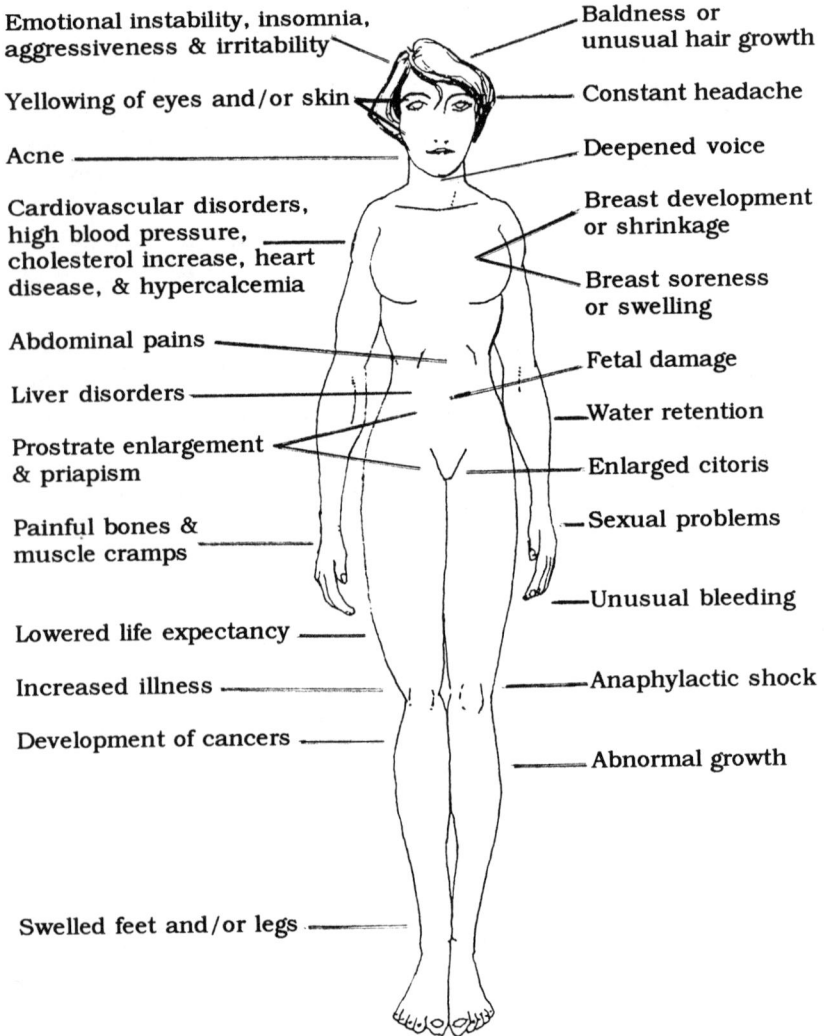

# "Drugs and Beyond"

Emotional instability, insomnia, aggressiveness & irritability

Yellowing of eyes and/or skin

Acne

Cardiovascular disorders, high blood pressure, cholesterol increase, heart disease, & hypercalcemia

Abdominal pains

Liver disorders

Prostrate enlargement & priapism

Painful bones & muscle cramps

Lowered life expectancy

Increased illness

Development of cancers

Swelled feet and/or legs

Baldness or unusual hair growth

Constant headache

Deepened voice

Breast development or shrinkage

Breast soreness or swelling

Fetal damage

Water retention

Enlarged citoris

Sexual problems

Unusual bleeding

Anaphylactic shock

Abnormal growth

Adverse effects and problem areas associated with short and long term use of
## Anabolic Steroids

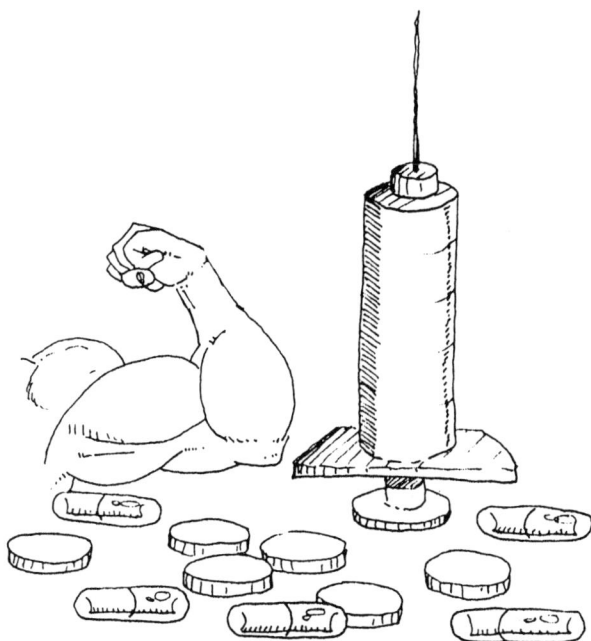

# OTHER DRUGS

**ANABOLIC STEROIDS** - are related to testosterone, a male sex hormone and are used to help build muscle tissues for increased skeletal muscle mass and strength and to improve athletic abilities.

Although they have many athletic uses, they are also used to rebuild tissues that have become weak due to injury or illness.

**Derivatives:** nandrolone, oxandrolone, oxymetholone, stanozolol.

**Brand Name: *Nandrolone*** - Anabolin, Anabolin LA-100, Androlone, Androlone 50, Androlone D, Deca-Durabolin, Durabolin, Hybolin Decanoate, Hybolin-Improved, Kabolin, Nandrobolic, Nandrobolic L.A., Neo-Durabolic; ***Oxandrolone*** - Anavar; ***Oxymetholone*** - Anadrol, Anapolon 50; ***Stanozolol*** - Winstrol.

# "Drugs and Beyond"

**Street Names:** roids.

**Medical Advantages:** are used to treat certain types of cancer, some rare conditions such as heredity angioedema (a reaction characterized by large, well - defined swellings, of sudden onset, in the skin, larynx (voice box), and other areas), to help rebuild tissues that have become weak due to serious illness or injury, and the growth hormone is used to treat pituitary dwarfism, to increase height and size and it will increase the use of lipid metabolism as an energy source; i.e.: cholesterol.

**Illegal Applications:** using this type of drug to build the body bigger and faster than one normally could as to qualify into an Olympic sport or sold on the street for profit.

**Appearance And Methods Of Use:** taken orally as tablets or (Nandrolone) by injection.

**Behavioral Characteristics:** drop in grades, increased illness, loss of personal possessions (sold to buy drugs), change of friends, mood swings, loss of interest in former goals, difficulty in concentrating and unusual borrowing of money. Also see "Short Term and Long Term Effects" for further evidence of abuse.

**Short Term Effects:** feeling of well-being and increased energy. Typical use results in increased doses over a number of weeks, causing tissue growth, rapid weight gain, water and oil retention, aggressive behavior and growth of male sex characteristics, cholesterol increase, fetal damage, edema, jaundice, liver tumors, priapism (prolonged painful erections), prostate enlargement, sterility, swelling of feet or lower legs, yellowing of eyes and/or skin, aggressive, combative behavior, abdominal or stomach pains, painful bones, chills, dark colored urine, fever, feeling of discomfort, anaphylactic shock (from injections), black, tarry or light colored stools, breast development, soreness or swelling in males, diarrhea, depression, fatigue, frequent urge to urinate, abdominal or stomach fullness, constant headache, hypercalcemia, impotence, higher risk of bodily injury, insomnia, kidney stones, muscle cramps, purple- or red - colored spots on the body or inside the mouth, sexual problems, unexplained darkening of the skin and weight loss, halitosis (constant bad breath), unusual bleeding, weight gain, vomiting of blood, hives, high blood pressure, kidney disorders, listlessness, nose rash, septic shock (blood poisoning from injections), sore tongue, urination problems and unnatural hair growth, especially in women.

**Long Term Effects:** may include cardiovascular complications, liver disorders, violence, cancer, heart disease, hirsutism (hairiness in women; irreversible), lowered life expectancy, increased risk of coronary artery disease, baldness, stunting of growth and male characteristics in females.

**Tolerance and Dependence:** tolerance and dependence are not developed with extended use of anabolic steroids, although they do produce symptoms of irritability and depression when use is discontinued. These symptoms may lead the user to continue the use of anabolic steroids and use may become a habit.

### Helpful Natural Treatments:

*Vitamins:* A, B, B complex, B1, B2, B3, B5, B6, B9, B12, Choline, C, Pangamic acid, Sodium ascorbate (buffered vitamin C), D, E and K.
*Minerals:* Calcium, Chromium, Iron, Magnesium (chelated form), Manganese, Selenium and Zinc.
*Aminos:* L-Glutathione, L-Lithium carbonate & L-Phenylalanine.
*Foods:* dark green leaves, flax, hemp seed, pumpkin seed, soy bean and walnut.
*Herbs:* Astragalus, Cowslip, Echinacea, Hops, Licorice Root, Lobelia, Milk Thistle, Ginseng, Golden Seal, and Valerian Root.
*Also:* Red Spearmint. This herb can help to safely alleviate restlessness associated with withdrawal symptoms.

If a person is serious about body building, a good diet and nutritional supplements should be sought as an alternative to steroids. The following is one example that can help to achieve this goal.

Arginine. Arginine or L-Arginine is an amino acid which is necessary for the normal function of the pituitary gland. Males, especially, need arginine since seminal fluids contain as much as 80 percent arginine and a deficiency could lead to infertility.

Although Arginine is not allowed to be sold in pure form in Canada, it is available in combinations and works best when is found with L-Ornithine, as they compliment each other.

The best foods arginine is found in are: all protein-rich foods, brown rice, carob, chocolate, gelatine desserts, nuts, oatmeal, popcorn, raisins, sunflower and sesame seeds and whole-wheat bread.

**ANTIHISTAMINES** - are drugs which block the action of histamine, a substance released by the body in some allergic reactions. They are effective in reducing symptoms such as itching, congestion, runny nose, sneezing and skin conditions.

Only recently did illicit use of these drugs come about because of its principal sedative side effect. Because of the often unpleasant side effects and capability to overdose, they are best left alone.

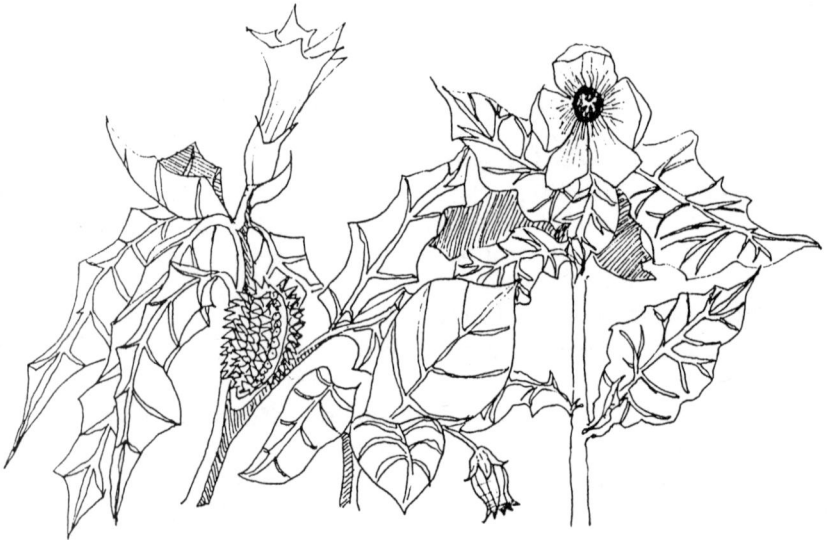

**JIMSON WEED - BELLADONNA - HEMBANE**

**ANTISPASMODIC / ANTICHOLINERGIC AGENTS** - are alkaloids found in belladonna (a deadly nightshade), Jimsonweed (datura), henbane (Hyoscyamus niger) and mandragora (mandrake). Found in these plants are the alkaloids atropine, scopolamine and hyoscyamine. The latter two alkaloids are so similar to atropine that the three are often referred to as "the belladonna alkaloids." Atropine, scopolamine, and hyoscyamine are among many synthetic agents used mainly for their antispasmodic and anticholinergic properties.

In surgery, some are given by injection before anesthesia to relax the person and to lessen secretions, such as saliva.

Some of these agents are also used to treat poisoning caused by medicine, certain types of mushrooms, and poisoning by nerve gases or organic phosphorous pesticides. Anticholinergic drugs can be used to treat painful menstruation, to prevent urination during sleep, and for runny nose.

Atropine is often used to dilate the pupils of the eye, to relax the stomach and intestines for certain types of examinations and is sometimes injected to relieve cramps or spasms of the stomach, intestines, and bladder. When used for the eyes, it is done so before some eye examinations, before and after eye surgery, and to treat certain eye conditions.

Atropine is quite milder than scopolamine or hyoscyamine, which are not used as often in medicine as atropine, although, all three are sometimes combined in tranquilizing medications. During surgery and anesthesia, atropine, hyoscyamine and scopolamine are used to keep the heart rate normal.

If large enough doses of atropine are taken, sensations of flying, disorientation and hallucination are consequences that some find enjoyable, among others. Some deterrents to the illicit use of atropine are: delirium; excitement; hot, dry skin and mucous membranes; blurred vision; confusion; rapid pulse and respiration; paralysis and coma. Brain damage and death can occur with very heavy doses.

Angel's Trumpet is an atropinelike hallucinogen which grows wild in several Gulf and Southeastern states. The flowers are eaten or made into a tea to produce a state similar to that of atropine (when atropine is taken in large doses) caused by scopolamine, the principal alkaloid in this plant and the most potent in its class.

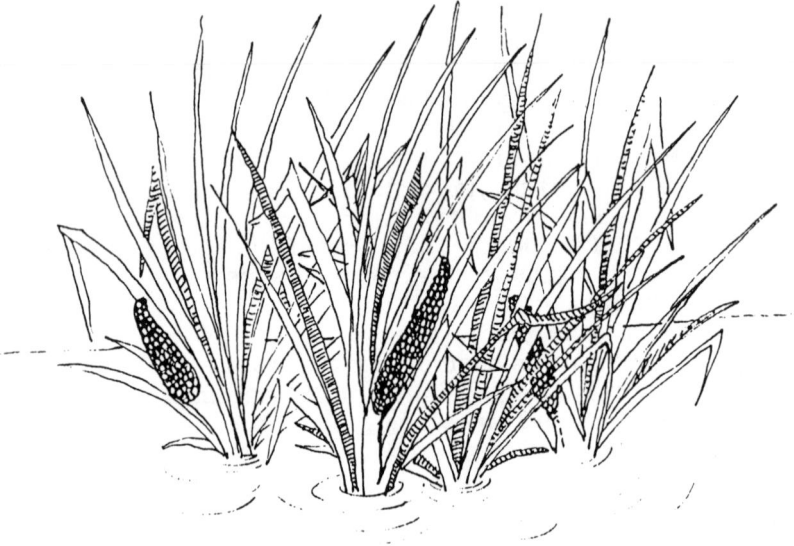

## SWEET FLAG

**ASARONE** - this drug comes from the roots of sweet flag and the Asarum species and is related to mescaline and amphetamines. Action of this drug can be as a stimulant, sedative and hallucinogen at the same time.

**CAT (Methcathinone)** - is a highly addictive stimulant which is easily made from such common household and industrial chemicals as paint thinner and drain cleaner. The key ingredient is ephedrine, which is sold as a stimulant and for nasal congestion due to hay fever and other allergies, low blood pressure, narcolepsy, and certain types of mental disorders. CAT is extremely hard on the body and leaves its addicts looking as if they were dead.

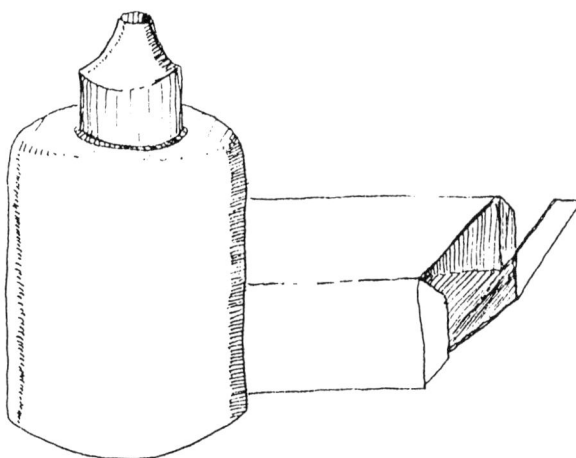

## DECONGESTANTS

**DECONGESTANTS** - are drugs, substances or procedures that relieve congestion or swelling; especially of the nasal passages. Phenylephrine is the most common ingredient in over-the-counter decongestants and is also a mild stimulant. Oral decongestants raise heart rate and blood pressure and may increase pressure in the eye. When taken in high doses, hallucinations, dizziness or lightheadedness, mood or mental changes, nervousness or restlessness and nausea and vomiting are some of the effects that may occur.

**DEXAMYL or DRINAMYL** - is a dextroamphetamine - barbiturate combination which has been given the street name "Purple Hearts" and can have serious side effects if abused; not excluding death.

**DITRAN (Piperidyl Benzilate)** - is an hallucinogen. It distorts ones perception of time, color, space and hearing.
    Experimentation has revealed subjects becoming totally insensate to the outside environment, incoherent and immobile.

**EPHEDRINE** - is a CNS stimulant, an adrenergic bronchodilator (a medicine which opens up the air passages of the lungs), and is chemically very similar to epinephrine (adrenaline).

Ephedrine can be used to stop bleeding when applied directly to the skin; to relieve congestion from allergies; in the treatment of narcolepsy; in emergency treatment of allergic reactions; and to treat minor dermatological problems, such as skin rashes; itching; hives; and swelling of the lips, tongue, eyelids and inside of the nose. It has also been used to treat overdoses of alcohol, barbiturates and opiates.

**HARMINE** - is obtained from the seeds of the Peganum Harmala, a plant from the Middle East, and is an hallucinogen, CNS stimulant and serotonin antagonist. Small oral doses can produce mental excitement and euphoria and sometimes the user will enter a dreamlike state in which everything is perceived to be moving in wavelike patterns. If taken intravenously or in larger doses, hallucinations can be produced. The common reaction for harmine users is they become very passive and they tend to relax.

**MORNING GLORY SEEDS (Ololiuqui) AND HAWAIIAN WOODROSE SEEDS** - are used as intoxicants and as hallucinogens by Central and South American Indians. They are used in rituals as a means of communicating with the supernatural. The seeds can be eaten whole, ground and eaten or filtered (percolated) and drunk as a beverage.

D-lysergic acid amide is one of several compounds which make up the psychedelic action of this naturally occurring agent and was taken to replace LSD when the drug was scarce.

When ingested, the immediate effects included nausea, headache, dilated pupils, vomiting, increased blood pressure, and sleepiness.

**NUTMEG AND MACE** - the actual nutmeg nut, used as a garnish for eggnog, and the outer shell, mace, have been used to produce an hallucinogenic trip. Intense hallucinations, both visual and tactile, can be produced, but so much is needed, it is extremely hard on the body. The effects on the body include: abdominal spasm, constipation, drowsiness, insomnia, strain on the kidneys, and tachycardia. The main discouragement for further administration is the vomiting and long term kidney pain that follow once the trip is completed.

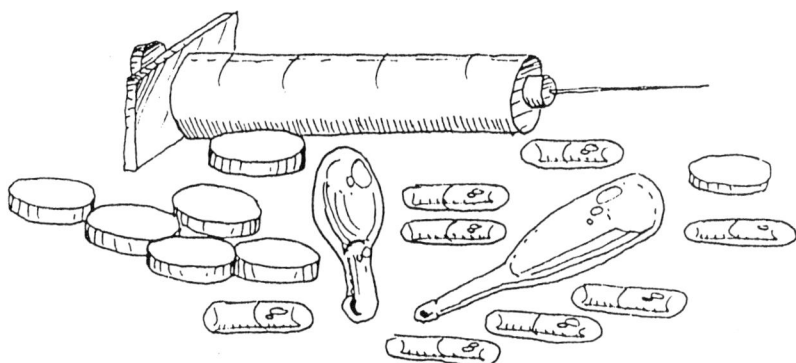

## PARALDEHYDE

**PARALDEHYDE** - is used to treat certain convulsive disorders, in medicine where barbiturates cannot be tolerated and has been used in the treatment of alcoholism and of nervous and mental conditions to calm and relax them and to produce sleep. Paral (a brand name for paraldehyde) is addictive, considered to be more intoxicating than barbiturates and alcohol, and the severity of withdrawal is slightly greater than that of alcohol.

**PMA** - is of the hallucinogens and is found as beige, white, or pink powder. It has effects similar to that of LSD's, coupled with a racing pulse, high blood pressure, labored breathing, high fever, muscle spasms and vomiting.

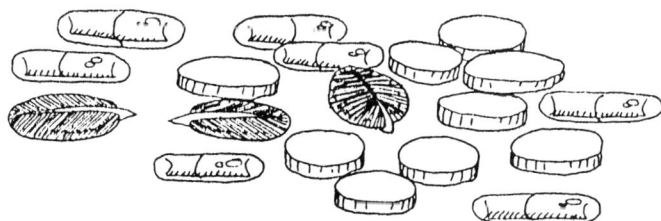

## STRYCHNINE

**STRYCHNINE** - is a drug which, in the 1800's, was used to increase circulation and stimulate the heart. The most common place to see strychnine now is in rodent poisons, although it is sometimes used to revive people overdosed on CNS depressants and reversibly, depressants are used to revive a strychnine overdosed person.

Overdose on strychnine is extremely probable (symptoms being convulsions, photosensitivity, stiffness of the face and neck and muscle spasms) and should be treated with utmost caution.

*Note:* If overdose is suspected, seek medical help immediately.

**YOHIMBINE HYDROCHLORIDE** - is a stimulant and mild hallucinogen and is sometimes used as an aphrodisiac. Being either snorted or eaten, it produces subtle perceptual and mood changes and a series of spinal rushes and shivers. Medicinally, it is used to treat breathing disorders due to heart problems.

### Helpful Natural Treatments For This Section:

*Vitamins:* A, B, B complex, B1, B2, B5, B6, B9, B12, Choline, C, Pangamic acid, Sodium ascorbate (buffered vitamin C), D, E and K.

*Minerals:* Calcium, Chromium, Iron, Magnesium (chelated form), Manganese, Selenium and Zinc.

*Aminos:* L-Glutathione, L-Lithium carbonate & L-Phenylalanine.

*Foods:* dark green leaves, flax, hemp seed, pumpkin seed, soy bean and walnut.

*Herbs:* Astragalus, Cowslip, Echinacea, Hops, Licorice Root, Lobelia, Milk Thistle, Ginseng, Golden Seal, and Valerian Root.

*Also:* Red Spearmint. This herb can help to safely alleviate restlessness associated with withdrawal symptoms.

# *Helpful Natural Treatments Which Aid In Recovering From Drug Addictions*

If a person is dependent on any of the drugs listed in the book and wishes to discontinue its/their use, medical help must first be sought as withdrawal symptoms can be life threatening.

The following chart is designed to help a dependent person discontinue the use of the drug(s) he/she is using, possibly without having to take synthetic drugs to slowly alleviate withdrawal symptoms. It is not designed to be prescriptive or diagnostic, but is intended to give natural alternatives to conventional recovery practices.

The suggested alternatives can be forwarded to the medical physician and may be used alone or in combination with the treatments recommended by the physician.

Throughout the book we have placed only the most general natural treatments for the individual misused drugs and have included natural supplements, plus a general use of common herbs, aminos, minerals, vitamins, enzymes and foods.

The intent of this chart is to put you in touch with the herbs which will be most beneficial in natural therapy of one's specific problem.

Some of the herbs listed throughout this book can be deadly if wrongly used and should only be used according to the doses prescribed by the manufacturer. Please read the label warnings carefully.

# HERBAL ALTERNATIVES

| Name | Source | Effects |
|---|---|---|
| American Mistletoe | *Phoradendron flavescens* | Mild Sedative. |
| Anise | *Pimpinella anisum* | Stimulant. |
| Angelica | *Angelica archangelica* | Stimulant. |
| Bird's-foot Trefoil | *Lotus corniculatis* | Antispasmodic and mild sedative. |
| Black Birch Bark & Oil | *Betula lenta* | Analgesic. |
| Black Cohosh | *Cimicifuga racemosa* | Antispasmodic, relaxant and mild sedative. |
| Black Haw | *Viburnum prunifolium* | Sedative. |

| Methods Of Use | Use To Replace... | Toxicity |
|---|---|---|
| Leaves are brewed into a tea. | Benzodiazepines, antihistamines, and all other mild depressants. | American Mistletoe is listed as unsafe by the U.S. Food and Drug Administration. |
| Brewed into a tea. | Caffeine; in larger doses. | None. |
| Brewed into a tea or purchased as capsules. | Tobacco and caffeine. | Angelica should not be used by pregnant women as it discharges menstrual fluids or diabetics as it may cause weakness. |
| Brewed into a tea. | Benzodiazepines, antihistamines, and all other mild depressants. | The flowers and leaves of the Bird's-foot Trefoil contain cyanide, which can be fatal. |
| Oil is added to food and eaten. | Pain associated with withdrawal symptoms. | None. |
| Brewed into a tea or used as poultice for minor pains. | Benzodiazepines, antihistamines, and all other mild depressants. | Large doses may cause miscarriage and symptoms of poisoning. |
| Brewed into a tea. | Benzodiazepines, antihistamines, and all other mild depressants. | None. |

# HERBAL ALTERNATIVES

| Name | Source | Effects |
|------|--------|---------|
| Boneset | Eupatorium perfoliatum | Stimulant. |
| Bugleweed | Lycopus virginicus | Sedative. |
| Button Snakeroot | Eryngium yuccifolium | Stimulant and in larger doses, serves as a nauseant. |
| California Laurel | Umbellularia californica | Analgesic. |
| California Poppy | Eschscholzia californica | Analgesic and sedative. |
| Cankerroot | Coptis groenlandica | Mild sedative. |
| Cardamom; Also Cardamum or Cardamon | Elettaria cardamomum | Stimulant. |
| Cardinal Flower | Lobelia cardinalis | Is both sedative and stimulant. |

| Methods Of Use | Use To Replace... | Toxicity |
|---|---|---|
| Tops of the Boneset are brewed into a tea or purchased as capsules. | Caffeine. | None. |
| Brewed into a tea or purchased as capsules. | Benzodiazepines, antihistamines, and all other mild depressants. | None. |
| Brewed into a tea or chewed fresh. | Amphetamines or tobacco. | None. |
| Leaves are dried and made into a tea or chewed fresh. | Pain associated with withdrawal symptoms. | None. |
| Eaten, brewed into a tea or smoked. | Benzodiazepines, antihistamines, and all other mild depressants. | None. |
| Rhizomes and roots are eaten fresh or brewed into a tea. | Benzodiazepines, antihistamines, and all other mild depressants. | None. |
| Fruit and seeds brewed into a tea or dried and used as a spice. | Caffeine or tobacco. | None. |
| Eaten fresh or brewed into a tea. | Tobacco or alcohol. | None. |

# HERBAL ALTERNATIVES

| Name | Source | Effects |
|------|--------|---------|
| Catnip | *Nepeta cataria* | Mild sedative. |
| Celery | *Apium graveolens* | Mild sedative. |
| Chamomile | *Matricaria chamomilla* | Sedative. |
| Cinnamon | *Cinnomomum zeylanicum* | Stimulant. |
| Cloves | *Caryophyllus aromaticus* | Stimulant. |
| Couch Grass | *Agropyron repens* | None. Use as a caffeine-free coffee substitute. |
| Cumin | *Cuminum cyminum* | Stimulant. |
| Damiana | *Turnera Diffusa* | Mild stimulant. |
| English Holly | *Ilex aquifolium* | Mild sedative. |

| Methods Of Use | Use To Replace... | Toxicity |
|---|---|---|
| Brewed into a tea or smoked. | Benzodiazepines, antihistamines, and mild depressants. | None. |
| Seeds eaten with food or brewed into a tea. | Benzodiazepines, antihistamines, and all other mild depressants. | None. |
| Flowers brewed into a tea or purchased as capsules. | Benzodiazepines, antihistamines, and mild depressants. | None. |
| Smoked or dried and eaten. | Tobacco or caffeine. | None. |
| Brewed into a tea, eaten fresh or purchased as capsules or oil. | Caffeine or tobacco. | None. |
| Drank as coffee substitute. | Coffee. | None. |
| Used topically and as a spice. | Caffeine. | None. |
| Leaves are smoked or purchased as capsules. | Tobacco. | None. |
| Brewed into a tea. | Benzodiazepines, antihistamines, and mild depressants. | The seeds are poisonous and when eaten, will cause vomiting and severe emptying of the bowels. |

# HERBAL ALTERNATIVES

| Name | Source | Effects |
|------|--------|---------|
| **European Cowslip** | *Primula veris* | Antispasmodic, mild analgesic, and mild sedative. |
| **European Mistletoe** | *Viscum album* | Stimulant. |
| **Fo-Ti** | *Polygonum multiflorum* | Stimulant. |
| **Garden Heliotrope** | *Valeriana officinalis* | Antispasmodic and a strong sedative. |
| **German Chamomile** | *Matricaria chamomilla* | Antispasmodic and a sedative . |
| **Ginger** | *Zingiberis officinalis* | Stimulant. |
| **Ginseng** | **American** *(Panax quinquefolius);* **Korean** *(Panax Ginseng);* **Siberian** *(Eleuther-ococcus Senticosus)* | Stimulant. |
| **Heather** | *Calluna vulgaris* | Mild sedative. |

| Methods Of Use | Use To Replace... | Toxicity |
|---|---|---|
| Brewed into a tea. | Benzodiazepines, antihistamines, and all other mild depressants. | None. |
| Brewed into a tea or purchased as capsules or fluid extract. | Caffeine. | The berries are poisonous and Mistletoe, in large doses, can cause heart problems. |
| Brewed into a tea or purchased as capsules or extract. | Caffeine. | None. |
| Roots and rhizomes are brewed into a tea. | Barbiturates, benzodiazepines, antihistamines, and mild depressants. | None. |
| Brewed into a tea. | Benzodiazepines, antihistamines, and all other mild depressants. | None. |
| Brewed into a tea or purchased as capsules or extract. | Caffeine. | None. |
| Dried and chewed or powdered and brewed into a tea. | Amphetamines or tobacco. | Some people have found Korean, or Panax, Ginseng too stimulating, but it is not harmful. |
| Brewed into a tea. | Benzodiazepines, antihistamines, and all other mild depressants. | None. |

# HERBAL ALTERNATIVES

| Name | Source | Effects |
|------|--------|---------|
| Henbane | Hyoscyamus niger | Strong narcotic and hallucinogen. |
| Hop | Humulus lupulus | Sedative. |
| Horehound | Marrubium vulgare | Mild sedative and laxative in large doses. |
| Hydrangea | Hydrangea paniculata | Stimulant. |
| Indian Tobacco | Lobelia inflata | Euphoriant and muscle relaxant. |
| Jimsonweed (Thorn Apple) | Datura Strammonium | Strong hallucinogen. |
| Juniper | Juniper macrodopa | Strong hallucinogen. |

| Methods Of Use | Use To Replace... | Toxicity |
|---|---|---|
| Brewed into a tea. | PCP, cocaine, crack, and the opiates. | In large doses, A Slow And Painful death will result! Also it is listed as unsafe by the U.S. Food and Drug Administration |
| Brewed into a tea. | Benzodiazepines, antihistamines, and mild depressants. | None. |
| Brewed into a tea in large quantities. | Benzodiazepines, antihistamines, and all other mild depressants. | None. |
| Smoked. | Tobacco. | Unknown. |
| Smoked or brewed into a tea. | Marijuana. | Indian Tobacco - is listed as being unsafe by the U.S. Food and Drug Administration. Also, large doses can be fatal! |
| Brewed into a tea. | Other hallucinogens and alcohol. | Jimsonweed Indian Tobacco has been declared poisonous by the U.S. Food and Drug Administration. Also, in large doses, a slow and painful death will result! |
| Smoked. | Other hallucinogens and alcohol. | Juniper should not be used by pregnant women or people who have kidney disease. |

# HERBAL ALTERNATIVES

| Name | Source | Effects |
|------|--------|---------|
| **Kava** (**Kavakava**) | *Piper methysticum* | Mild hallucinogen. |
| **Lady's-slipper** | *Cypripedium calceolus* | Sedative. |
| **Lavender Cotton** | *Santolina chamaecyparissus* | Stimulant. |
| **Lemon Balm** | *Melissa officinalis* | Sedative. |
| **Madagascar Periwinkle** | *Catharanthus roseus* | Hallucinogen. |
| **Mate** | *Ilex paragueyensis* | Stimulant. |
| **Mormon Tea** | *Ephedra nevadensis* | Stimulant. |
| **Oats** | *Avena sativa* | Antidepressant. |
| **Passion-flower** | *Passiflora incarnata* | Analgesic and sedative properties. |
| **Peach** | *Amygdalus persica* | Sedative. |

| Methods Of Use | Use To Replace... | Toxicity |
|---|---|---|
| Smoked or brewed into a tea. | Marijuana. | Long term use can cause liver damage and if smoked, lung disorders may result. |
| Boiled extract of the roots is eaten with food. | Benzodiazepines, antihistamines, and other mild depressants. | None. |
| Seeds and flowers brewed into a tea. | Tobacco and caffeine. | None. |
| Leaves. | Mild depressants. | None. |
| Smoked or brewed into a tea. | Marijuana and its derivatives. | May be poisonous in large doses. |
| Brewed into a tea. | Tobacco. | May be poisonous in large doses. |
| Brewed into a tea. | Tobacco and caffeine. | None. |
| Eaten in large quantities. | Some antidepressant drugs. | None. |
| Dried fruits and flowers eaten or brewed into a tea. | Marijuana and its derivatives, benzodiazepines, antihistamines, and mild depressants. | None. |
| Leaves and bark are brewed into a tea or purchased as capsules. | Benzodiazepines, antihistamines, and all other mild depressants. | Pregnant women should avoid this herb. |

# HERBAL ALTERNATIVES

| Name | Source | Effects |
|------|--------|---------|
| **Prickly Ash** | *Zanthoxylum americanum* | Stimulant. |
| **Prickly Lettuce** | *Lactuca scariola* | Mild narcotic analgesic. |
| **Prickly Poppy** | *Argemone mexicana* | Narcotic analgesic. |
| **Rauwolfia (Snakeroot)** | *Rauvolfia serpentina* | Tranqilizer and hypotensive agent. |
| **Red Poppy** | *Papaver rhoeas* | Mild Sedative. |
| **Rosemary** | *Rosarinus officinalis* | Stimulant. |
| **Skullcap** | *Scutellaria lateriflora* | Antispasmodic and sedative. |
| **Spearmint** | *Mentha spicata* | Is a stimulant and alleviates restlessness associated with withdrawal symptoms. |

| *Methods Of Use* | *Use To Replace...* | *Toxicity* |
|---|---|---|
| Eaten freah (bark) or brewed into a tea. | Tobacco and caffeine. | None. |
| Smoked or brewed into a tea. | Opium. | None. |
| Smoked as an euphoriant. | Opium. | The seeds and leaves are poisonous when taken internally which can be harmful |
| The root is eaten fresh or can brewed into a tea. | Benzodiazepines, antihistamines, and mild depressants. | It is a major source of *reserpine* and it can cause edema, bad dreams and other disorders which may lead to suicidal tendencies. |
| Smoked or brewed into a tea. | Benzodiazepines, antihistamines, and all other mild depressants. | None. |
| Leaves and flowers are brewed into a tea or purchased as capsules or oil. | Caffeine. | Do not exceed three cups of tea daily or take undiluted oil orally. |
| Brewed into a tea. | Benzodiazepines, antihistamines, and all other mild depressants. | May cause stupor, confusion, giddiness and twitching in large doses. |
| Leaves eaten fresh or brewed into a tea. | Use in association with common withdrawal practices. | None. |

# HERBAL ALTERNATIVES

| Name | Source | Effects |
|------|--------|---------|
| Wild Cherry Bark | Prunus serotina | Sedative. |
| Wild Yam | Dioscorea villosa | Steroidlike properties. |
| Wormwood | Artemisia absinthium | Narcotic analgesic. |

| Methods Of Use | Use To Replace... | Toxicity |
|---|---|---|
| The inner bark is brewed into a tea or purchased as capsules or extract. | Benzodiazepines, antihistamines, and mild depressants. | None. |
| The roots can be brewed into a tea. | Steroids. | Has contraceptive properties so should not be used by pregnant women |
| Smoked or brewed into a tea. | Opium. | Wormwood is declared as being unsafe by the U.S. Food and Drug Administration. |

## "Drugs and Beyond"

## QUESTIONS AND ANSWERS FOR PARENTS AND TEENAGERS.

This is a test which can help parents and teenagers talk and learn about drugs. To make it easier, parents should take the test first and then the teenager.

## QUESTIONS

*1*. I don' t need to discuss drugs with my parents. *T  F*

*2*. Alcohol is a drug. *T  F*

*3*. Music is more enjoyable if I have taken drugs. *T  F*

*4*. Drugs have no harmful effects on a persons health. *T  F*

*5*. If, at a party, someone offered me drugs, I would accept. *T  F*

*6*. I will discuss drugs with my children. *T  F*

*7*. I don' t need to know about drugs. *T  F*

*8*. Drugs should become legal. *Yes  No*

*9*. The use of cocaine is worse than the use of alcohol. *T  F*

*10*. The use of any drug will lead to addiction. *T  F*

# ANSWERS

**1. F.** Discussion about drugs in the family is very helpful to make everyone aware about what drugs are and what they do. It will also make it easier to talk about a problem that may exist or which may arise involving drugs with one or more family members.

**2. T.** Although alcohol is legal, it is a drug.

**3. F.** Each drug has its own effect to the senses. When someone is high on drugs, it isn't that the music sounds better it is that the music sounds different. The music can be pleasing in this state, but it still is not the way the artist would have liked it to sound, therefore, it is not better.

**4. F.** Drugs can have a severe effect on the users health. Although not every drug has the same severity as the next, it is true that each drug is potentially harmful. These effects can vary from raising ones heartbeat to causing the user to vomit, have severe diarrhea or even cause a heart attack or coma.

**5.** Though the expected answer is false, there is no right or wrong answer to this question since this more for discussion purposes.

**6.** Again, this question is designed for discussion purposes. It is well advised, though, to discuss drugs with your children since it will make it that much easier for future discussion.

**7. F.** Everyone should know whatever they can about drugs so if they are ever approached, they can decide on the basis of what they know rather than what they don' t know.

**8.** There is no right or wrong answer as this is a discussion question.

**9.** This is not really a true / false question, but rather a question to make the point that all drugs are potentially addictive. An addictive drug can lead to abuse and abuse can lead to the body slowly deteriorating because of physical damage and mental instability.

**10. F.** Drugs have there place in our world just like everything else. Under the right conditions, drugs are no more addictive than any other chemical that enters our body every day, but the key here is controlled conditions.

# Commonly Used Street Terms

**A Fix** - one injection of narcotics, usually heroin.

**"A Head"** - an habitual user of the amphetamines.

**A Hit** - street slang for a dose of drugs.

**A La Canona** - abrupt withdrawal from heroin without the use of any treatment or medications; Peurto Rican slang.

**A-Bomb** - a joint dusted with opium or heroin.

**Acapulco Gold** - marijuana of gold color, high potency, and said to be grown in the area of Acapulco, Mexico.

**Acid** - slang for LSD.

**Acid Freak** - one who uses LSD and whose behavior is bizzarely affected.

**Acid Head** - is someone who uses LSD frequently.

**Acid Rock** - music which is usually listened to by LSD users and is characterized by being loud, electronic, frenetic and fast.

**Ames** - small glass vials of amyl nitrate.

**Angel Dust** - slang for PCP (phencyclidine).

**Angel Off** - arresting the buyers from a dealer who is being watched.

**Anywhere** - possessing or holding drugs.

**Baby** - marijuana.

**Backwards** - tranquilizers used to bring someone back from acid or speed.

**Bador** - hallucinogenic seed from the morning glory plant; Aztec slang.

**Bad Seed** - peyote.

**Bad Trip** - having an unpleasant experience with a drug; usually the hallucinogens.

**Bag** - packet of drugs; the measured amount of a drug indicated by the price; one's lifestyle.

**Bagman** - a drug dealer.

**Bale** - a pound of marijuana.

**Bam** - an amphetamine to be injected or taken orally.

**Banana Smoking** - a previous fad in which a person smoked the inner peelings of the banana to get high, although it has not been proven to be effective.

**Bang** - to inject drugs intravenously.

**Bank Bandit Pills** - barbiturates or other sedative pills.

**Bar** - a solid block of marijuana stuck together with honey or sugar water.

**B-Bombs** - benzedrine inhalers which were removed from the market in 1949.

**Beast or The Beast** - LSD.

**Beat** - to cheat or rob someone of money or goods; a round, line or district regularly traversed, as by a sentry, policeman or reporter.

**Bee** - a box or bag of marijuana.

**Belly Habit** - heroin withdrawal pains subjectively centered in the stomach.

**Bennies** - benzedrine pills.

**Bent** - slang for being intoxicated from a drug or drugs.

**Bernies** - cocaine.

**Bhang** - the marijuana plant and the drink made with marijuana used to produce psychotropic effects; the word originating from India.

**Big Bags** - $5 to $10 bags of heroin; the price may vary.

**Big Bloke** - cocaine.

**Big Chief** - peyote or mescaline.

**Big "D"** - LSD.

**Big Man** - the distributor of wholesale ilicit drugs to other dealers.

**Big Supplier** - the distributor of wholesale ilicit drugs to other dealers.

**Bindle** - small folded paper containing heroin.

**Bingle** - drug dealer.

**Black Beauties** - biamphetamine capsules.

**Black Gunion** - extra thick, potent, dark, gummy marijuana.

**Black Pills** - pellets of opium.

**Black Russian** - dark-colored, very potent hashish.

# "Drugs and Beyond"

**Blank** - a container of white powder sold as heroin, but was not.

**Blast** - to smoke a drug.

**Blast Party** - a group of people gathered together to smoke drugs, usually marijuana.

**Blockbusters** - white and yellow striped pills of barbiturates.

**Blotter Acid** - LSD on porous paper.

**Blow** - cocaine; to smoke marijuana; to snort cocaine or heroin; to miss a vein while administering it intravenously.

**Blow Snow** - to snort cocaine.

**Blow Your Mind** - to alter one's conciousness drastically, usually with drugs.

**Blow Your Mind Roulette** - a game played with barbiturates and amphetamines.

**Blue Acid** - LSD.

**Bluebirds** - amytal sodium capsules.

**Blue Heavens** - amytal sodium capsules.

**Blue Velvets** - a combination of terpin hydrate elixir, codeine and tripelennamine.

**Blue Liner** - is a fine - line syringe developed specifically for insulin users which is now commonly used among drug users.

**Blue Heavens** - slang for barbiturates.

**Body Drugs** - drugs which can become physically dependent.

**Body Trip** - drug experience which seems physical rather than mental.

**Bogue** - withdrawal from physical-dependence-producing drugs.

**Bolsa** - bag of heroin.

**Bombed Out** - slang for being intoxicated from a drug or drugs.

**Bomber** - a big or thickly rolled joint.

**Bong** - a type of pipe used to smoke marijuana.

**Boo** - marijuana.

**To Boot** - to buy alcohol for an underaged person.

**Booting** - injecting heroin a little at a time in order to prolong the initial pleasurable effects.

**Bouncing Powder** - cocaine.

**Boxed** - being intoxicated from a drug or drugs.

**Brain Ticklers** - amphetamine or barbiturate pills.

**Bread** - money.

**Brick** - a pressed block of marijuana, hashish, heroin or opium, usually in pounds or kilograms.

**Brownies** - amphetamines, especially dexedrine capsules; brownies baked with marijuana, hashish or the oils.

**Buzz** - slang term for a high or a drug induced euphoria.

**Brick** - a pressed block of marijuana, hashish, opium, or heroin usually in pounds or kilograms.

**Bum Bend** - a bad trip.

**Bum Kicks** - troubled, worried or depressed.

**Bummer** - a bad trip.

**Bundle** - a package of twenty-five $5 bags of heroin stacked together.

**Burese** - cocaine.

**Burn** - to cheat or steal.

**Burning** - smoking marijuana.

**Burn Out** - to overexploit or overuse a drug, person or place so that it is no longer desirable to continue with it.

**Bush** - marijuana.

**Business Man's Trip** - DMT, because it has such a short duration, it can be taken at a lunch break and not interupt with the activities for the rest of the working day.

**Bust** - to arrest or to be arrested by the police.

**Button** - small disks from the peyote cactus made by cutting the top into thin pieces.

**Buy** - to purchase drugs.

**Buzz** - moderate high from any drug without hallucinations.

**C.** - cocaine.

**Caapi** - hallucenogenic tea made from the vine, banisteriopsis.

**Ca-Ca** - counterfeit or very-poor-quality drugs.

**Canadian Black** - a variety of marijuana grown in Canada.

# *"Drugs and Beyond"*

**Candy Man** - a drug dealer.

**Cannabis** - a family of plants called marijuana; the proper name is *Cannabis Sativa*.

**Cap** - the capsule of a drug.

**Carry** - to have drugs on one's person.

**Cartwheels** - amphetamine tablets.

**Catnip** - strong-smelling herb sometimes sold as marijuana to unsuspecting buyers.

**Chalk** - amphetamine tablets.

**Charas** - resin taken from the flowering tops of the female hemp or cannabis plants in India; also known as hashish.

**Charles** - cocaine.

**Charlie** - a dollar.

**Chasing the Bag** - hustling for, or being dependent on, heroin.

**Chasing the Dragon** - inhaling the fumes of a heroin and barbiturate mixture which is placed in tinfoil and heated over a flame.

**Chief** - LSD.

**Chill** - to ignore or to refuse a deal with someone, in relation to drugs; the word is also used to tell someone to calm down.

**Chipping** - using heroin irregularly to avoid physical dependence.

**Chota** - an informer (Puerto Rico).

**Chronic** - slang for a person addicted to the hallucinogens.

**Cibas** - Glutethamide.

**Clean** - free from suspicion; not having drugs in one's possession; marijuana with the seeds taken out of it.

**Coasting** - a drowsy, nodding state of a heroin user just after a recent injection.

**Cocktail** - an ordinary cigarette used to smoke the end of a joint; made by removing a bit of tobacco from the plain cigarette.

**Coke** - slang for cocaine.

**Coke Head** - an habitual user of cocaine.

**Cold Turkey** - sudden withdrawal from chronic narcotic use without supplementary drug treatment.

**Collar** - to be arrested by the police.

**Colombian** - a type of marijuana grown in Colombia and area.

**Comatose** - a person who has fallen into a deep sleep after overindulging themselves in the hallucinogens; usually marijuana.

**Come Down or Coming Down** - the gradual loss of effect of a drug.

**Connect** - to find a source, or to buy, drugs.

**Contact** - a drug supplier or dealer.

**Contact Habit** - experiencing the effects of physical dependence on a drug by constantly associating with those who use it and are dependent on it.

**Cook** - to heat a mixture of heroin and water until the heroin is dissolved.

**Cooker** - a small metal container or apparatus where a cocaine and water mixture are heated; i.e.- a spoon.

**Cop** - to connect; to score; to buy narcotics; a police officer.

**Co-Pilot** - one who stays with a person who has taken a powerful drug (usually LSD) to make sure the person is alright and to help if the user has a bad trip.

**Corrine** - cocaine.

**Courage Pills** - barbiturates and other sedative pills.

**Crack** - smokable form of cocaine, a freebase crystalline alkaloid.

**Crank** - street name for some amphetamines.

**Crap** - low-quality drugs.

**Crashing** - withdrawal from amphetamines (going from high to extreme low); to go or to fall asleep; to come down from a stimulating drug.

**Creep** - a person using heroin who does not engage in risky activities to pay for the drugs; an eery or perverted person may be reffered to as a creep.

**Croke** - a mixture of a form of speed, methamphetamine and cocaine, snorted or injected.

**Crossroads** - amphetamine tablets.

# "Drugs and Beyond"

**Crutch** - anything to hold the last bit of a joint so it can be completely smoked; an excuse given as not to admit that one is addicted to a drug, i.e.- *amphetamines are my crutch to make it through the day.*

**Crystal** - street name for PCP, speed, amphetamines, methedrine or desoxyn.

**Cut** - the dilution of a drug with another substance to make more quantity.

**D.** - doriden (glutethimide).

**Dabbling** - irregular use of physically dependent drugs as to not become dependent.

**Dagga** - marijuana (South Africa).

**Datura** - jimson weed; devil's weed; found in Mexico, the United States, South America and India. It has psychotropic properties.

**Deadly Nightshade** - belladonna.

**Deal** - to buy or sell drugs.

**Dealer** - one who sells drugs illicitly.

**Dealer's Band** - a rubberband placed around the wrist to secure packets of drugs so that if the wrist is flipped violently, the drugs will fall from the wrist.

**Deck** - folded paper or glassine envelope which contains drugs (usually cocaine or heroin).

**Deeda** - LSD.

**Dexies** - dexedrine tablets.

**Dime** - $10.

**Dirty** - a person who, or a place which, possesses drugs.

**Djamba** - marijuana.

**Djomba** - marijuana; also called diamba, liamba, lianda and macona in Central Africa.

**DMT** - short for N, N-dimethyltrypyamine, a fast acting hallucenogenic drug with a short duration period.

**Dogie** - heroin; also called doojee or duji.

**Dollies** - dolophine pills.

**Dolophine** - methadone; a synthetic opiate slightly more potent than morphine, and with a much longer duration of action.

**Dom** - STP.

**DOM** - STP; 2,5-dimethoxy-4-methylamphetamine; an hallucenogenic drug about 100 times as potent as mescaline and 1/3 as potent as LSD.

**Dope** - slang for marijuana and any other drug which will produce a change in mental state

**Dope Fiend** - a term used by physically dependant users to defiantly describe themselves.

**Do or Doing** - a replacement word for "use", i.e.- he's doing weed.

**Do Up** - to inject a drug intravenously.

**Downers** - slang for barbiturates, tranquilizers and sedative drugs; also down, downs or downies.

**Down Trip** - a boring or depressing experience.

**Dragged** - to be frightened or hysterical after using a drug.

**Dreamer** - morphine.

**Dried Out** - detoxified; no longer physically dependant on a drug or drugs; a dealer or user who has run out of drugs.

**Drop** - to take any drug orally.

**Dropper** - a medicine dropper used as a syringe to take drugs by injecting.

**Druggies** - people who experiment with all sorts of drugs; regular or chronic users of a drug or drugs.

**Dube , Duber or Duby** - marijuana.

**Dummy or Dummies** - counterfeit heroin or cocaine; also called blank, crap, garbage, lemonade or shit.

**Dusted** - is a term used when a powdered drug is added to another drug.

**Duster** - a cigarette made of tobacco, mint leaves, marijuana or parsley sprinkled with PCP; cocaine.

**Dynamite** - a very potent drug; cocaine and heroin mixed together.

**Eight - ball** - one eighth ounce of cocaine.

**Eighth** - one-eighth ounce of a drug.

**Electric** - containing an hallucenogenic drug.

# "Drugs and Beyond"

**Electric Kool-Aid** - a liquid beverage made with Kool-Aid and an hallucenogenic drug.

**Embalao** - being strongly addicted or strung out; Puerto Rican slang.

**Enchaioui** - a man who has centered his life around marijuana; Arabic slang.

**Epena** - hallucenogenic snuff made from the bark of trees and used by Indians in Brazil.

**Esrar** - marijuana; Turkish.

**Explorers Club** - a group of illicit LSD users.

**F-40's** - secobarbital.

**Factory** - a place where drugs are produced, diluted or cleaned for sale.

**Falling Out** - falling asleep under the influence of a drug.

**Fatty** - a big or thickly rolled joint.

**Feds** - Federal Bureau of Narcotics agents.

**Fit** - to severly crave a drug; to need a drug as soon as possible, usually to rid the body of unwanted withdrawal symptoms.

**Five Cent Paper** - a $5 bag of heroin.

**Five Dollar Bag** - bag of heroin sold for $5 and containing 5 grains from 0 to 80 percent pure heroin.

**Fives** - tablets containing 5 mg. of a drug.

**Fix** - to take a drug intravenously.

**Flagging** - is when the user of a drug injects a needle through the skin and checks for blood in the syringe, showing that he/she has hit a vein.

**Flake** - cocaine.

**Flashback** - the recurrence of an hallucination originally experienced under the influence of an hallucinogenic drug.

**Flashing** - glue sniffing.

**Flea Powder** - a very poor drug.

**Flip Out** - state of fear and loss of control produced by a drug; fear brought on by some external influence, usually when under the influence of a drug, but may be due to a flashback.

**Floating** - under the influence of a drug, usually the hallucinogens.

**Flower Power** - believing in the power of love rather than force.

**Flush** - sudden onset of euphoria from a drug.

**Flying** - under the influence of a drug.

**Flying Saucers** - a variety of the morning glory plant.

**Footballs** - diamphetamine pills; dilaudid.

**Forwards** - amphetamine pills.

**Freak** - a person who prefers a certain drug over the rest and uses it regularly, usually because of the bizarre effects it has on that person; a person who acts differently from the rest of society in an unacceptable way.

**Freaking Freely** - random, spontaneous behavior, usually influenced by an hallucinogenic drug.

**Freak-Out** - a panic reaction due to the effects of a drug or experience.

**Freebase** - removing the salts and other additives from cocaine which will produce a from that is smokable.

**Freebasing** - smoking crack; a smokable form of cocaine.

**Frisco-Speedball** - heroin, cocaine and LSD taken together.

**Friut Salad** - a game which consists of each participant consuming one of each pill from a medicine cabinet.

**Full Moon** - a large peyote chunk greater than 4 inches in diameter.

**Fuzz** - police officers, especially narcotics officers.

**Gage (Gauge)** - marijuana.

**Gammon** - one microgram of LSD.

**Ganja** - a potent form of marijuana obtained from the flowering tops and leaves of the plant; Jamaican; also spelled ganga, gunja or gunga.

**Gangster** - marijuana.

**Gangster Pills** - barbiturate or other sedative pills.

**Gaping** - withdrawal symptoms.

**Garbage** - very poor quality drugs.

# "Drugs and Beyond"

**G.B.** - goofball; barbiturates.

**Gee Head** - a person who is physically dependant on paregoric.

**Get Down** - use heroin.

**Get Off** - to experience a change in consciousness or mental state as a result of the intake of drugs

**Get On** - to experience drugs, or a drug, for the first time.

**Ghanja** - active principle of marijuana in a highly concentrated form.

**Ghost** - LSD.

**Giggle Weed** - marijuana; magic mushrooms.

**Girl** - cocaine.

**Glass** - smokable chunks of speed.

**Globetrotter** - a person who goes to various drug dealers looking for the best drugs, usually looking for heroin.

**Glow** - under the influence of a drug or drugs.

**Going Down** - going well; the process of being arrested for trafficing (selling) drugs.

**Going High** - a seemingly endless state of intoxication.

**Gold Dust** - cocaine.

**Golden Leaf** - a form of marijuana called Acapulco Gold.

**Goods** - any kind of drug, usually a large amount to be distributed by a dealer.

**Good Stuff** - the best drugs of any kind.

**Goof Balls** - slang for barbiturates.

**Gorilla Pills** - barbiturates and other sedative pills.

**Goof Balls** - slang for barbiturates.

**Grass** - slang for marijuana.

**Gravy** - a mixture of blood taken from a vein and heroin which must be reheated because it has coagulated and then injected back into the body through a vein.

**Greasy or Greaseball** - a person who will make no effort to obtain money for drugs, yet will always sit in on a session.

**Greasy Junkie** - a passive person who is physically dependent on heroin, yet makes not effort to obtain money for drugs.

**Green** - the cheapest form of marijuana; money.

**Grefa** - marijuana; also greta, grifa and griffe.

**Guide** - a person who guides another through an hallucinogenic experience.

**Guru** - a person who guides another through an hallucinogenic experience.

**H.** - heroin.

**Half Load** - fifteen packages of heroin wrapped together for resale.

**Hand to Hand** - the transfer of drugs at the point of sale.

**Haraz** - police officer; Puerto Rican slang.

**Hard Stuff, Hard Drugs or Hard Narcotics** - derivatives of opium, usually heroin; cocaine; sometimes hallucinogens.

**Harry** - heroin.

**Hash(ish)** - a form of marijuana made from the resins of the flowering tops of the cannabis sativa plant and its resins.

**Hash Oil** - a form of marijuana extracted from cannabis sativa.

**Hawk** - LSD.

**Hay** - marijuana.

**H-Caps** - gelatin capsules of heroin.

**Head** - a person who uses drugs.

**Head Drugs** - drugs which appear to affect a person's mind and not the body.

**Head Shops** - where the sale of drug related items are available.

**Hearts** - amphetamines.

**Heat** - police officers.

**Heaven Dust** - cocaine; PCP.

**Heavenly Blue** - a variety of morning glory seeds which have hallucinogenic properties.

**Hemp** - marijuana; the tough, strong fiber from the Cannabis Sativa plant, used for cloth, paper, ropes and cords.

**Henry** - heroin.

**Her** - cocaine.

**Herb** - marijuana.

# "Drugs and Beyond"

**High** - widely used term for intoxication.

**Him** - heroin.

**Hit** - a single unit of measure in relation to the drug being administered; to inject intravenously.

**Hold** - to have drugs on one's person.

**Honey Oil** - is the purest form of the marijuana resin oils.

**Hookah** - a pipe used for smoking marijuana.

**Hooked** - physically dependent on a drug or drugs.

**Hoot** - a single inhalation of smoke from a joint.

**Hop** - opium.

**Hophead** - a person physically dependent on heroin or opium.

**Horse** - heroin.

**Hot Boxing** - making the air in an enclosed space dense with the smoke from marijuana so it can be continuously inhaled to continue the "high" until the air becomes less dense and discontinues its effects.

**Hot Knifing** - the placing of an hallucinogen onto a knife to be heated and the smoke inhaled for the purpose of getting "high."

**Hot Shot** - an injection that is supposed to be heroin, but is actually poison.

**Hungry Croaker** - a doctor who will prescribe drugs to a physically dependent person for money.

**Hustling** - getting money for drugs by stealing, prostitution, pawning items off, etc.; deliberately lying for personal gain, usually for drugs.

**Ice** - smokable form of crystal methamphetamine.

**Ice Cream Habit** - moderate or infrequent use of drugs producing physical dependence.

**Idiot Pills** - barbiturates or other sedative pills.

**Indian Hay** - marijuana.

**Indian Hemp** - marijuana.

**Inhale** - inspire; to draw in the breath; to breathe in the smoke or fumes of a drug or abused substance.

**Into** - using or paying special attention to something, especially drugs.

***In Transit*** - on an LSD trip.

***J. or Jay*** - short for joint.

***Jag*** - a prolonged state of consciousness caused by a drug.

***Jammed Up*** - having taken an overdose.

***Jerk Off*** - injecting a small amount of heroin at a time to prolong the initial euphoria.

***Joint*** - a hand-rolled marijuana cigarette.

***Jones*** - physical dependence on a drug or drugs.

***Joy Juice*** - chloral hydrate; appetizers; tonics.

***Joypop*** - irregular use of heroin to avoid physical dependence, yet will experience euphoria.

***Juanita*** - marijuana.

***Juice*** - any alcoholic beverage.

***Juice-Head*** - an alcoholic; a person who prefers alcoholic beverages.

***Junk*** - heroin.

***Junkie*** - a heroin addict or a person addicted to other narcotics.

***Kava*** - a mild psychotropic drink drunk by the people of New Guinea.

***Key (Ki)*** - a kilogram of a drug; Kilo.

***Kick (The Habit)*** - to withdraw from physical dependence of a drug or drugs.

***Kicks*** - a pleasurable or enjoyable experience.

***Kick The Habit On The Elevator*** - refers to a person who is physically dependent ever-so-slightly that they could withdraw from the use of the drug very easily.

***Kilo*** - a kilogram of a drug; key.

***Kilter*** - marijuana.

***L.*** - LSD.

***Lady Snow*** - cocaine.

***Leapers*** - amphetamines.

***Lemonade*** - very poor quality drugs.

***Lid*** - one ounce of marijuana.

# "Drugs and Beyond"

**Lid Poppers** - amphetamines.

**Life** - the life of a person with a characteristic pattern of revolving around drugs.

**Light Stuff** - marijuana and other hallucinogenic drugs which produce no physical dependence.

**Light Up** - the act of starting or lighting a joint.

**Line** - the vein used to inject drugs.

**Load** - about 25 to 30 packets of heroin held to gether with an elastic band for delivery.

**Loco** - marijuana.

**LSD or LSD-25** - D-lysergic acid diethylamide tartrate 25; acid; a strong hallucinogenic drug with strong psychedelic properties.

**Lush** - a heavy drinker or an alcoholic.

**Magic** - containing an hallucenogenic drug.

**Magic Mushrooms** - strong hallucinogenic mushrooms which contain psylocibin and/or psilocin and possess strong psychedelic properties.

**Mainline** - injecting a drug into a vein (to shoot up); the vein used to inject drugs.

**Majoon (majoun)** - hash(ish) produced in the middle east.

**Making A Croaker For A Reader** - bribing a doctor to illegally prescribe drugs for ilicit use.

**Man** - a police officer; a word used quite often to refer to the person being spoken to.

**Mary** - morphine.

**Mary Jane** - marijuana; also Mary Ann, Mary Warner and Mary Weaver.

**Matchbox** - a small matchbox full of marijuana for sale.

**MDA** - 3-methoxy-4,5 methlenedioxyamphetamine; a phenyliso-propylamine, which means that it has chemical similarities to amphetamine and properties similar to mescaline.

**Mellow Yellow** - the slang term denoting banana smoking.

**Mesc** - mescaline; the alkaloid in the peyote cactus which produces most of the hallucinogenic effects.

**Methamphetamine** - a very powerful amphetamine; also called methedrine or desoxyn.

**Meth Freak** - a person who uses methamphetamine habitually; also known as a speed freak.

**Mexican Brown or Mexican Green** - a grade of marijuana.

**Mexican Locoweed** - marijuana.

**Mexican Mushroom** - a type of hallucinogenic mushroom.

**Microdot** - a tiny tablet of LSD.

**Microgram** - one millionth of a gram.

**Mike** - one microgram of a drug, especially LSD.

**Milk Sugar (Mannite)** - a substance used to cut a powdered drug to produce more of it.

**Milligram** - one thousandth of a gram.

**Mind Detergent** - LSD.

**Mind Trippers** - people who use drugs to explore their minds.

**Miss Emma** - morphine.

**M.J.** - marijuana.

**Mojo** - heroin; cocaine; morphine.

**Monkey** - a person physically dependent on a drug.

**Moon** - a peyote cactus top; cake; bulk hash(ish).

**Mooch or Moocher** - a person who consistantly recieves drugs without paying for them.

**Morning Shot** - an injection taken as soon as one wakes up from a sleep.

**Morph** - morphine.

**Mota** - marijuana.

**Mother** - a drug dealer.

**Mu** - marijuana.

**Muggles** - marijuana joints.

**Nabbed** - to be discovered; to be arrested by the police.

**Nail** - an hypodermic needle used to inject drugs; also called a spike.

**Narc** - a narcotics police officer; also called narco fuzz or narco.

**Natch or On The Natch** - not using drugs.

# "Drugs and Beyond"

**Needle Park** - a place used for shooting up or injecting drugs.

**Nemish or Nemmies** - nembutal capsules.

**Nickel** - $5.

**Nodding** - drowsy; dreamy; a dozing state following the injection of heroin or the other opiates characterized by the person's head falling or lowering forward and slowly jerking up and down.

**O.** - opium.

**O.D. or O.D.'d** - overdosed.

**Ololiuqui** - the Aztec name for morning glory seeds.

**On** - a replacement word for "using", i.e.- "What's he on?" or "He's on acid man."

**On The Needle** - injecting drugs.

**Opiate or Opioid** - a derivative of, or relating to, opium.

**Outfit** - equipment used for injecting drugs.

**Overjolt** - overdose.

**O.Z.** - one ounce.

**P.** - peyote.

**Panama Red** - a type of marijuana.

**Paper** - a piece of paper folded as a packet containing drugs.

**Peaches** - benzedrine tablets.

**Pearls** - small glass vials of amyl nitrate.

**Pellets** - capsules of LSD.

**People** - sometimes used to refer to police officers.

**Pep Pills** - amphetamines.

**Peyote** - Lophophora Williamsii; a cactus and hallucinogenic drug which is found in southern parts of the United States.

**Phenos** - barbiturates, especially phenobarbital and seconal.

**Picked Up** - smoked marijuana; purchased drugs.

**Piece** - a measure or part of a quantity of drugs; a gun.

**Pill or Pill Head** - one who uses barbiturates or amphetamines; barbiturates or amphetamines.

**Pin or Pinner** - a small, thin marijuana joint.

**Pinks** - seconal.

**Pinned** - constricted, usually referring to the pupils of the eyes.

**Plant** - a hiding place for drugs; to put on another's person as to not be caught by the police; marijuana.

**Poison** - heroin; fentanyl.

**Poison People** - those physically dependent to heroin or fentanyl.

**Poke** - a single inhalation of a marijuana joint.

**Pop** - to take drugs orally is to *pop* them; to inject a drug by purposely missing the vein so the drug can slowly disslove through the muscle tissues, producing a longer duration of effects; also known as skin popping.

**Popped** - haven taken drugs orally or by skin popping; being discovered or arrested by the police.

**Pot** - slang for marijuana.

**Pot Head** - is a person who uses "pot" or marijuana regularly.

**Potlikker** - the tea or a person who drinks the tea made by brewing marijuana seeds and stems.

**Potsville** - using marijuana; a place where marijuana is either grown or sold in abundance; the latter can also be called Potville.

**Primo** - very good quality drugs, especially marijuana.

**Psychedelic Art** - art which tries to mimic the hallucinogenic effects induced by hallucinogenic drugs.

**Psychotropic** - mind-changing; altering conciousness.

**Purple Hearts** - luminal tablets; a combination of amphetamines and barbiturates.

**Pusher** - a drug dealer; a person who tries to pursuade others into trying a certain drug or drugs to get them addicted, so he/she can sell to them and make a greater profit.

**Quarter Bag** - one-quarter ounce of a drug; a bag which sells for $25.

**Quill** - a folded matchbook cover used to snort drugs.

**Rainbow** - a tuinal capsule.

**Rainy Day Woman** - a marijuana joint.

**Rap** - to talk.

**Rat** - someone who gives information to the police or other figure of authority.

# "Drugs and Beyond"

**Reader** - a prescription for drugs.

**Reds and Blues** - tuinal capsules.

**Red Birds** - seconal capsules.

**Red Devils** - seconal capsules.

**Red Dirt Marijuana** - marijuana that grows in the wild.

**Reds** - seconal capsules.

**Reefer** - a marijuana joint.

**Rig** - hypodermic equipment.

**Righteous Bush** - marijuana.

**Ripped** - intoxicated, usually alcohol.

**Roach** - the small end of a marijuana joint that is left after most of the cigarette has been smoked.

**Roach Clip** - a device used to hold the roach.

**Rock Houses** - fortified dwellings where crack or rock cocaine is sold.

**Rolling Buzz** - a moderate high from a drug that continues after the intake of the drug has stopped.

**Rolling Papers** - cigarette papers used to make a marijuana joint.

**Root** - a marijuana joint.

**Roses** - benzedrine tablets.

**Run** - a period of time in which a person continually takes a drug without stopping, may last for hours or even for days depending on the type of drug; the purchasing of drugs.

**Rush** - the short-term state of exhilaration at the beginning of a high.

**Sacred Mushrooms** - magic mushrooms.

**Salt Shot** - a misconception that, when a person has overdosed on one of the opiates an injection of water and salt will revive them.

**Scag** - heroin.

**Scales** - used to weigh drug quantities for sale purposes.

**Scars** - needle marks which cause scars on the body.

**Schmack (Smack)** - heroin; cocaine; can also be any other drug.

**Schmeck** - heroin.

**Scissors** - marijuana.

**Scoff** - to take orally; to eat food.

**Scoop** - folded matchbook cover used to snort drugs.

**Score** - to successfully find a connection to drugs.

**Scratch** - to be physically dependent on drugs.

**Scrip or Script** - a prescription for drugs.

**Seccy or Seggy** - seconal capsules.

**Shit** - marijuana; vey poor quality drugs.

**Shlook** - a single inhalation of smoke from a joint.

**Shooting Gallery** - a place where people gather to inject drugs.

**Shoot Up** - to inject drugs.

**Sick** - withdrawal symptoms, especially heroin.

**Sizzle** - drugs which are on one's person.

**Skid Bag** - a bag containing highly diluted heroin.

**Skin** - cigarette paper used to roll a joint.

**Skinning** - skin popping.

**Skin Popping** - injecting a drug under the skin, not in a vein.

**Sleep Walker** - a person who is physically dependent on heroin.

**Smack** - heroin; a smacker is a person who uses heroin.

**Smoking Stones** - paraphernalia used to hold a marijuana joint while smoking.

**Snappers** - small glass vials of amyl nitrate.

**Sniffing** - inhaling a drug through the nose.

**Snop** - marijuana.

**Snort** - inhaling a drug through the nose.

**Snow** - cocaine.

**Source** - a supplier of drugs.

**Spaced** - intoxicated; also called spaced out.

**Sparkle Plentics** - amphetamines.

**Speed** - amphetamines, methamphetamine or methedrine.

**Speedball** - an injected mixture of heroin and cocaine.

# "Drugs and Beyond"

**Speed Freak** - one who takes amphetamines often.

**Spike** - an hypodermic needle.

**Splash** - amphetamines.

**Split** - to go; run away; to divide into equal parts.

**Splits** - tranquilizers.

**Spoon** - usually 1/16 of an ounce of heroin; an eating utencil used to heat, mix and/or dilute drugs.

**Star Dust** - cocaine.

**Stash** - any container or place used to store a drug; hidden drugs.

**Steamboat** - inhaling smoke through certain paraphernalia to make the smoke cool.

**Stick** - a marijuana joint.

**Stoned** - slang for being intoxicated.

**Stone Addict** - a person who is physically dependent on drugs of a very potent nature.

**Stool or Stoolie** - someone who gives information to the police or other figure of authority.

**STP** - DOM; an hallucinogenic drug with exceptionally long effects, lasting from 36 to 72 hours.

**Straight** - not using drugs.

**Strung or Strung Out** - physically dependent on a drug.

**Stuff** - drugs, especially heroin.

**Supergrass** - slang for marijuana treated with PCP.

**Super Pot** - very potent marijuana.

**Sunshine** - LSD as an orange tablet.

**Sweet Lucy** - marijuana.

**Swingman** - drug dealer or pusher.

**Tabs** - short for tablets.

**Tall** - intoxicated or euphoric.

**Tapita** - a bottle cap used for cooking heroin.

**Taste** - a small amount of a drug, usually given as a gift.

**Tea** - marijuana.

**Tea Bag** - the state of smoking marijuana.

**Tea Head** - a person who uses marijuana regularly.

**Tecata** - heroin.

**Ten-Cent Pistol** - a heroin bag which contains poison.

**Texas Tea** - marijuana or a black marijuana oil.

**THC** - tetrahydrocannabinol, the main ingredient in marijuana and its derivatives which is responsible for its effects.

**Thrusters** - amphetamine pills.

**Thumb** - a fat marijuana joint.

**Ticket** - LSD.

**Tin** - a small amount of opium.

**Tingle** - a rush; the first onset of effects brought on by a drug.

**TMA** - a synthetic hallucinogen of greater potency than mescaline, but being very similar in terms of its effects.

**Toak or Toke** - slang for an inhalation of marijuana.

**Toke Pipes** - short-stemmed pipes through which marijuana smoke is inhaled.

**Tooies** - tuinal capsules.

**Tools** - paraphernalia.

**Topi** - peyote cactus.

**Torn Up** - intoxicated.

**Toss Out** - faking withdrawal symptoms to a doctor in order to obtain a prescription for the drug.

**Tracked Up** - having needle marks on the skin resulting from repeated injection of drugs.

**Tracks** - scars on the skin resulting from repeated injection of drugs.

**Travel Agent** - a dealer who supplies LSD.

**Trip** - effects of a hallucinogen or psychedelic.

**Trips** - drugs which produce hallucinogenic effects.

**Turn On To** - to introduce someone to a drugs or experience for the first time.

**Twenty-Five** - LSD-25, which is the proper abbreviation for the LSD used by people who take this drug.

# "Drugs and Beyond"

**Twist** - marijuana.

**Tying Up** - tying something to the upper arm so the veins will stand up making it easier to inject the drug.

**Up** - intoxicated.

**Upper** - an amphetamine pill.

**Up-Tight** - tense, worried, anxious.

**Using** - to take any drug.

**Vipe** - marijuana.

**Viper** - a marijuana smoker.

**Voyager** - a person under the influence of LSD.

**Wake-Up** - a person who is physically dependent on heroin and injects it the first thing in the morning.

**Waste** - destroy; throw away; to kill someone.

**Wasted** - to be severly intoxicated.

**Water Pipe** - paraphernalia used to smoke drugs (i.e.. marijuana) that filters the smoke through water.

**Weed** - slang for marijuana.

**Weeding Out** - smoking marijuana; quitting the use of marijuana.

**White Cross** - X-scored tablet, 15 to 20 mg. of methamphetamine.

**White Lady** - heroin; cocaine.

**White Light** - a wonderful experience gained through the use of hallucinogenic drugs under special conditions.

**White** - benzedrine pills.

**White Stuff** - heroin; cocaine.

**Wired** - highly stimulated, especially under the influence of a stimulant; carrying a microphone or other recorder to record exactly what is being said in a drug bust to be used in court as evidence.

**Wingoing** - physical withdrawal symptoms from drug dependence.

**Wings** - the first intravenous injection.

**Window Pane** - LSD in small squares of coated plastic or stiffened gel.

**Works** - implements needed to administer drugs through injection; spoon, syringe, tie off, container for mixing, filter and the drug or drugs.

**Wrap** - innocent looking covering for drugs.

**Yellow Jackets** - nembutal capsules.

**Yen** - withdrawal symptoms from physically addicting drugs.

**Zebra Hash** - is either morroccan or beige hash mixed with white powdered opium giving a zebra pattern.

**Zonked** - intoxicated.

**Zooming** - slang term used to describe the effects of psychedelic mushrooms.

# *Glossary*

**Abscess** - a circumscribed collection of pus appearing in acute or chronic, localized infection, and associated with tissue destruction and, frequently, swelling.

**Acute - 1.** acting keenly on the senses; sharp and severe. **2.** coming quickly to a turning point; brief and severe. **3.** threatening; critical.

**Addict** - a person who is a slave to a habit.

**Addiction** - physical dependence on a drug. Physical withdrawal symptoms may be experienced if use is stopped suddenly after taking the drug repeatedly.

**Administer** - to supply or provide with; apply, as a medicine or treatment.

**Adrenalin** - see Epinephrine.

**Agitation** - strong emotional disturbance.

**Alkaloid** - any one of many plant products distinguished by basic reactions, now restricted to heterocyclic nitrogen - containing and often complex structures possessing pharmacological activity; i.e., atropine, nicotine, caffeine, cocaine, etc.

**Amenable** - open to influence, suggestion, or advice.

**Amenorrhea** - absence or abnormal cessation of the menses.

**Amino Acid** - any one of a group of complex organic compounds of nitrogen, hydrogen, carbon, and oxygen that combine in various ways to form the proteins that make up living matter.

**Amnesia** - partial or total loss or impairment of memory.

**Anabolic** - relating to or promoting the process of assimilation of nutritive matter and its conversion into living substance. This includes synthetic processes and requires energy.

**Analgesia** - absence of the sence of pain without loss of conscious-ness

**Analgesic** - of or causing analgesia.

**Anaphylactic Shock** - a reaction including shock, difficulty breathing, itching and hives, convulsions and coma due to immediate and sometimes life - threatening allergic hypersensitivity.

**Androgen** - any of various hormones that control the development of masculine characteristics.

**Anesthetic** - a compound that reversibly depresses neuronal function, producing loss of ability to perceive pain and/or other sensations.

**Anesthetize** - to make (a person animal or area of the body) unable to feel pain, touch, cold or other sensation.

**Angel Dust** - slang for PCP (phencyclidine).

**Aneurysm** - a bulging of the wall of a blood vessel, usually caused by hardening of the arteries and high blood pressure.

**Angioedema** - a reaction characterized by large, well - defined swellings, of sudden onset, in the skin, larynx (voice box), and other areas.

**Anorexia** - loss of appetite.

**Anorexia Nervosa** - a personality disorder manifested by extreme aversion to food, usually occurring in young women, resulting in extreme weight loss, amenorrhea, and constitutional disorders.

**Antagonist** - something opposing or resisting the action of another; denoting certain muscles, drugs, etc., that tend to neutralize or impede the action or effect of others.

**Antibiotic** - any of a large class of substances, as penicillin, streptomycin, etc., having the power of destroying and arresting the growth of microorganisms.

**Antibody** - generally, any body or substance, soluble or cellular, which is evoked by the stimulus provided by the introduction of antigen and which reacts specifically with antigen in some demonstrable way.

**Anticholinergic** - a drug or substance which lessens muscle spasms in the bladder, lung and intestines, relaxes the iris muscles of the eye, decreases substances released by the somach, lung and mouth, decreases sweating and speeds up the heart.

**Anticonvulsant** - prevent or arrest convulsions.

**Antidepressant** - counteracting depression.

**Antigen** - any protein substance that causes the body to produce antibodies to counteract it. Bacteria are antigens. Antigens also include toxins and foreign blood cells.

# "Drugs and Beyond"

**Antihistamine** - any of certain drugs that neutralize the action of histamine in the treatment of hay fever, asthma, etc.

**Antisepsis** - prevention of infection by inhibiting the growth of infectious agents. See disinfection.

**Antiseptic** - relating to or capable of effecting antisepsis.

**Antispasmodic** - relieving or checking spasms.

**Antitussive** - relieving a cough.

**Anxiety** - a psychoanalysis apprehension of danger and dread accompanied by restlessness, tension, tachycardia, and dyspnea unattached to a clearly identifiable stimulus.

**Apathy** - absence of emotion; indifference; insensibility.

**Aphrodisiac** - substances which, when ingested, suggested, smelled or seen, cause arousing or increasing sexual desire or potency; i.e. - an aphrodisiac food, drug, odor, etc.

**Arrest** - a stoppage; an interference with or a checking of the regular course of a disease or symptom, or the performance of a function.

**Arrythmia** - loss of rhythm; denoting especially an irregularity of the heart beat.

**Artery** - any of the blood vessels or tubes that carry blood from the heart to all parts of the body.

**Arthritis** - inflammation of a joint or joints.

**Asarum Species** - any one of a genus of low, stemless herbs with dull brownish flowers and aromatic rootstock. The common american species is known as wild ginger or snakeroot.

**Asthma** - a chronic disease of the lungs that makes breathing difficult and causes coughing. Asthma is an allergy characterized by intermittent or continuous difficulty in breathing and a sense of constriction in the chest.

**Ataxia** - loss or failure of muscular coordination.

**Auditory** - pertaining to the sense of hearing or to the organs of hearing.

**Auricle** - the chamber of the heart that recieves the blood from the veins and forces it into a ventricle.

**Benign** - not dangerous to health; not malignant. Also see tumor.

**Blackout - 1.** partial or complete loss of vision and sometimes of consciousness due to decreased blood flow to the brain. **2.** inability to recall happenings or events which occured while intoxicated.

**Blood Pressure -** the pressure or tension of the blood within the arteries.

**Bong -** a type of pipe used to smoke marijuana.

**Breech Birth -** the birth of a child with the feet or buttocks first, rather than the head.

**Bronchi -** the two large main branches of the windpipe, one going to each lung.

**Bronchiole -** a very small branch of the bronchi.

**Cancer -** any of a group of often fatal diseases characterized by abnormal cellular growth and by malignancy.

**Candela -** a unit of measuring the strength or intensity of light, equal to 1/60 of the radiating power of one square centimeter of a black body at the temperature at which platinum solidifies (1772 degrees Celsius).

**Carboxyl -** a univalent radical, -COOH, existing in many organic acids, the hydrogen being replaceable by a basic element or radical, thus forming a salt.

**Cardiac - 1.** refering to the heart. **2.** referring to a person with heart disease. **3.** referring to the part of the stomach joined by the esophagus.

**Cardiac Arrest -** a sudden stop of the heart.

**Cardiac Fibrosis -** excessive growth of fibrous connective tissue in the heart.

**Cardiovascular -** of or affecting both the heart and the blood vessels, as hardening of the arteries and high blood pressure.

**Catalepsy -** a morbid state in which there is a waxy rigidity of the limbs that may be placed in various positions which will be maintained for a time; there is irresponsiveness to stimuli, the pulse and respiration are slow, and the skin is pale.

**Catatonia -** a syndrome characterized by periods of physical rigidity, negativism, excitement and stupor.

# "Drugs and Beyond"

**Catecholamine** - any one of a class of hormones, such as adrenalin, that acts upon the nerve cells.

**Cell** - the extremely small, basic unit of living matter of which all plants and animals are made.

**Cellular** - having to do with cells.

**Cerebral** - of the brain; of the cerebrum.

**Cerebrum** - The part of the human brain, certain areas of which control particular processes of thought and voluntary muscular movement; the brain as a whole.

**Chromosomes** - any one of the rod - shaped bodies found in the nucleus of a cell that appear when the cell divides. Chromosomes are derived from the parents and carry the genes that determine heredity, controlling the development of the organism and determining its nature.

**Chronic** - lasting a long time; lingering; long - continued.

**Circumscribed** - to put limits on; restrict.

**Clitoris** - a female organ; a small erectile organ at the upper part of the vulva, homologous to the penis.

**CNS** - central nervous system.

**CNS Depressant** - a substance, compound or chemical which depresses or slows down central nervous system activity.

**CNS Stimulant** - a substance, compound or chemical which stimulates or excites central nervous system activity.

**Coma** - a state of profound unconsciousness from which one cannot be roused.

**Compound** - a substance formed by chemical combination of two or more substances in definite proportions by weight.

**Constipation** - problems in passing stools (solid waste from the digestive tract which is released from the rectum).

**Constitutional Disorders** - disorders which relate to a system as a whole. i.e., central nervous system.

**Consumption** - the act of eating or drinking up.

**Contraction** - a shortening or increase in tension; denoting the normal function of muscular tissue.

**Convulsions** - a violent and involuntary contraction or series of contractions of the voluntary muscles.

**Coordination** - harmonious adjustment or working together.

**Copulation - 1.** sexual intercourse. **2.** a joining together; coupling.

**Corpuscles - 1.** any of the cells that form a large part of blood and lymph. Red corpuscles carry oxygen from the lungs to various parts of the body and remove carbon dioxide; some white corpuscles destroy disease germs. **2.** certain parts of the nervous system, such as skin nerve endings, that respond to pressure.

**Corticosteroid** - a steroid produced by the adrenal cortex; a corticoid containing steroid.

**Cortisone** - 17a, 21 - Dihydroxy - 4 - pregnene - 3, 11, 20 trione; a steroid isolated from the adrenal cortex that exhibits no biological activity until it is converted to hydrocortisone (cortisol); acts upon carbohydrate metabolism (glucorticoid), and influences the nutrition and growth of connective (collagenous) tissues.

**Cystic Fibrosis** - a hereditary disease of the pancreas, primarily beginning in childhood, characterized by excessive secretion from internal organs, malnutrition and accompanying respiratory infection.

**Delineate - 1.** to trace the outline of. **2.** to draw; sketch. **3.** to describe in words; portray.

**Delirium** - a temporary disorder of the mind that occurs during fevers, insanity, drunkenness, or a drugged state. Delirium is characterized by restlessness, excitement, strange ideas, and wild talk.

**Delusion** - a fixed belief maintained in spite of unquestionable evidence to the contrary. People with mental disorders, especially schizophrenics, often have delusions.

**Denote** - to be the sign of; indicate.

**Depersonalization** - a state in which a person loses the feeling of his/her own identity in relation to others in his/her family or peer group, or loses the feeling of his/her own reality.

**Depressant** - a drug or other substance that reduces the body's reactions and relaxes muscles.

# "Drugs and Beyond"

**Depression** - low spirits; sadness or gloominess. *Psychology.* A mental disorder characterized by prolonged feelings of despair and dejection, often accompanied by fatigue, headache, and other physical symptoms. *Medicine.* A lowering of the vital functions or powers, as by relaxing muscle tissue or depressing activity.

**Diagnosis** - the act or process of finding out what disease a person or animal has by examination and careful study of the symptoms.

**Diaphoresis** - perspiration; sweating.

**Diarrhea** or **Diarrhoea** - the condition of having too many and too loose movements of the bowels; usually, the stool is watery.

**Diastasis** (pl. **-ses**) - the rest period of the cardiac cycle, occuring between the diastole and the systole.

**Diastolic Blood Pressure** - the pressure caused by the regular expansion of the heart each time the cavities fill with blood. It alternates with the contraction (systole), the two making up the cardiac cycle that includes brief intervening periods of inactivity (diastases).

**Dilate** - to make larger or wider; expand; enlarge: *as the pupils do in the absence of light.*

**Disinfectant** - a substance or means used to destroy disease germs. Alcohol, Iodine, and carbolic acid are disinfectants. Heat is a disinfectant.

**Disinfection** - the destruction of disease germs.

**Disorder** - a sickness; disease.

**Disorientation** - loss of the sense of familiarity with one' surround-ings.

**Dissociation** - the seperation of an idea or feeling from the main stream of conciousness.

**Dissociative** - having to do with or causing dissociation.

**Dopamine** - a hormone produced by the adrenal glands that is essential to the normal nerve activity of the brain.

**Dosage** - the amount of medicine to be taken at one time.

**Duodenal Ulceration** - an ulceration in the wall of the duodenum, caused entirely or in part by the digestive action of gastric juice.

**Duodenum** - the first part of the small intestine, just below the stomach.

**Dwarfism** - the condition or character of being a dwarf; a generally underdeveloped condition of growth, especially in the bony tissues of the limbs.

**Dysphoria** - a condition characterized by restlessness, mental discomfort, and general unhappiness.

**Dyspnea** or **Dyspnoea** - difficult or labored breathing.

**Edema** - an abnormal accumulation of watery fluid in the tissues or cavities of the body, often causing visible swelling.

**Ejaculation** - 1. ejection; discharge. 2. Emission of seminal fluid.

**Elixir** - a medicine made of drugs or herbs mixed with alcohol and syrup.

**Emotion** - a strong feeling of any kind. Hate, fear, excitement, anger, love joy and grief are emotions.

**Emotional** - easily affected by emotion.

**Encopresis** - involuntary passage of feces; to achieve a bowel movement involuntarily.

**Enzyme** - a protein substance produced in living cells, that influences a chemical reaction within a plant or animal without being changed itself.

**Epilepsy** - a chronic disorder of the nervous system characterized by partial or complete loss of consciousness and sometimes convulsions. It is caused by a disturbance in the normal electric rhythm of the brain cells.

**Epinephrine** - Adrenalin; 3,4 - dihydroxy - a [methylaminomethyl] benzyl alcohol; a catecholamine neurohormone of the adrenal medulla that is the most potent stimulant (sympathomimetic) of adrenergic a- and b- receptors, resulting in increased heart rate and force of contraction, vasoconstriction or vasodilation, relaxation of the bronchiolar and intestinal smooth muscle, glycogenolysis, lipolysis, and other metabolic effects.

**Epistaxis** - a nosebleed; profuse bleeding from the nose.

**Erection** - the state of the penis, clitoris, or other bodily organ or part in which the erectile tissue has become distended (swelled out; expanded) and rigid (stiff; firm) by the accumulation of blood.

# "Drugs and Beyond"

**Ergot** - a disease of rye and other cereals in which the grains are replaced by blackish fungous growth.

**Euphoria**- a feeling of well-being or elation. A greater than normal sense of physical and emotional well-being. It is not based on reality; is out of proportion to its cause and is inappropriate to the situation. This is most commonly seen in some forms of mental disorders and in poisonous and drug-induced states.

**Expectorant** - causing or helping the discharge of phlegm.

**Extended Release,** - a drug made in such a way that its effects will last longer than the origional or normal form.

**Fatigue** - a task or exertion producing weariness; exhaustion.

**Fibrosis** - excessive growth of fibrous connective tissue in an organ or part of the body.

**Fibrous** - made up of fibers; having fibers.

**Fixity** - fixed condition or quality; permanence; steadiness; firmness.

**Flashback** - the recurrence of a hallucination originally experienced under the influence of a hallucinogenic drug.

**Fluorocarbons** - any of a group of very stable compounds of carbon and chlorine used as solvents, lubricants, insulators, and refrigerants.

**Flush - 1.** to become red in the face through a rush of blood; blush. **2.** to glow or shine with reddish brightness.

**Freebasing** - smoking crack; a smokable form of cocaine.

**Ganja** - a potent form of marijuana obtained from the flowering tops and leaves of the plant. May also refer to marijuana in general.

**Gastritis** - inflammation of the stomach, especially of the mucous membrane.

**Gastrointestinal Disorders** - disorders having to do with the stomach and intestines.

**Glaucoma** - a disease of the eye, characterized by pressure within the eyeball, hardening of the eyeball, and gradual loss of sight. It is common in old age.

**Glucose** - a kind of sugar occurring in plant and animal tissues. Carbohydrate is present in the blood mainly in the form of glucose. Glucose is not as sweet as cane sugar.

**Glycogen** - a starchlike carbohydrate stored in the liver and other animal tissues. It is changed into glucose when the body needs energy.

**Glycogenolysis** - the hydrolysis of glycogen and glucose.

**Habit** - a tendency to act in a certain way.

**Habitual** - done by habit; caused by habit.

**Halitosis** - bad or offensive breath.

**Hallucinations** - a condition of seeing (visual), hearing (auditory), tasting, smelling, or touching (tactile) things that exist only in a persons imagination.

**Hangover** - a condition of headache, nausea, or other symptoms of distress, resulting from drinking too much alcoholic liquor, often occurring in the morning.

**Harmonious** - agreeing in feelings, ideas or actions; getting or working along well together.

**Hashish** - a form of marijuana made from the resins of the flowering tops of the cannabis sativa plant and its resins.

**Hash Oil** - a form of marijuana extracted from cannabis sativa.

**Hemoglobin** - a substance in the red corpuscles of the blood made up of iron and protein. It carries oxygen from the lungs to the tissues and some of the carbon dioxide from the tissues to the lungs.

**Hemorrhage** or **Haemorrhage** - a bleeding, either within the body or from the body surface; discharge of blood, especially a heavy discharge from a damaged blood vessel. A nosebleed is a mild hemorrhage.

**Herpes** - any one of various virus diseases causing spreading blisterlike blotches on the skin or mucous membrane, such as shingles and cold sores.

**High** - widely used term for intoxication.

**Hirsutism** - the inordinate (much too great) growth of hairs on the body.

**Histamine** - a white, crystalline substance, C5 H9 N3, found in animal tissues. It reduces blood pressure, has a contracting action on the uterus, and is released in allergic reactions.

# "Drugs and Beyond"

**Hives** - a condition in which the skin itches and shows raised patches of red; urticaria. It is caused by an allergy to some food or drug, or a reaction as to heat or light.

**Homologue** or **Homolog** - a homologous thing, organ, or part.

**Homologous - 1.** corresponding in position, proportion, value, structure, or other property. **2.** corresponding in type of structure and in origin but not necessarily in function or appearance. *The foreleg of a horse, the arm of a man, and the wing of a bird are homologous.*

**Honey Oil** - is the purest form of the marijuana resin oils.

**Hormone** - a substance formed in the endocrine glands, which enters the bloodstream and affects or controls the activity of some organ, or of cells or tissues. Adrenaline and insulin are hormones.

**Hyperactive** - overactive; abnormally active.

**Hypercalcemia** - an excessive amount of calcium in the blood.

**Hyperreflexia** - a condition in which the deep tendon reflexes are exaggerated.

**Hypersalivation** - an excess secretion of saliva. Also sialism; sialismus; salivation sialorrhea; sialosis.

**Hypertensive** - characterized by or suffering from abnormally increased blood pressure.

**Hypertonia** - extreme tension of the muscles and arteries.

**Hyporeflexia** - diminished or weakened reflexes.

**Hyposalivation** - lessened secretion of saliva; drymouth.

**Ice** - smokable form of crystal methamphetamine.

**Illicit / Illegal** - not permitted by law.

**Illusion** - an appearance or feeling that misleads because it is not real; thing that deceives by giving a false idea; misleading appearance.

**Immobile** - not moving; not changing; motionless.

**Impotence** - inability of the adult male to achieve an erection.

**Incoherent** - having or showing no logical connection of ideas.

**Incontinence** - lack of self control; lack of chastity (moral purity; decency; virtue).

**Indole** or **indol** - a white, crystalline chemical compound with an unpleasant odor, produced artificially by the reduction of indigo or by other forms of synthesis, and also formed within the intestines. It is used as a reagent and in making perfumes.

**Inhale** - inspire; to draw in the breath; to breathe in the smoke or fumes of a drug or abused substance.

**Inhibit** - to hold back; hinder or restrain; to slow the process of.

**Inhibitors** - **1.** a person or thing that inhibits. **2.** any substance that hinders or slows down a chemical reaction. **3.** a substance that inhibits the activity of an enzyme.

**Injection** - the act of forcing a liquid into the body with a syringe.

**Intoxicate** - **1.** to make drunk. **2.** poison.

**Illusion** - an appearance or feeling that misleads because it is not real; thing that deceives by giving a false idea; misleading appearance.

**Inhibition** - an idea, emotion, attitude, habit or inner force holding back or checking one's impulses, desires or the like.

**Insane** - not sane; mentally ill; crazy.

**Insensate** - without sensation; lifeless; inanimate; lack of feeling(s).

**Insomnia** - chronic inability to sleep or to remain asleep during the night.

**Intramuscular** - situated in or affecting the inside of a muscle.

**Intravenous** - situated in or affecting the inside of a vein.

**Intoxicate** - to make drunk; poison; inebriate.

**Invulnerable** - that cannot be hurt or wounded; safe from attack.

**IU** - abbreviation for International Unit.

**Jaundice** - an unhealthy bodily condition that causes yellowness of the skin, eyes, and body fluids, and disturbed vision; icterus. It is caused by too much bile in the blood. Jaundice is a symptom of some diseases and ailments, such as infectious hepatitis or gallstones.

**Lactation** - **1.** the secretion or formation of milk. **2.** the time during which a mother gives milk. **3.** the act of a suckling baby.

**Laryngitis** - inflamation of the mucous membrane lining the voice box (larynx), accompanied by swelling of the vocal cords with hoarseness or loss of voice.

**Lethargy - 1.** drowsy dullness; lack of energy; sluggish inactivity. **2.** a state of prolonged unconsciousness resembling deep sleep, from which the person can be aroused but immediately loses consciousness again.

**Libido - 1.** sexual energy or desire. **2.** the energy associated with instincts.

**Lipase** - any one of a class of enzymes occurring especially in the pancreatic and gastric juices and certain seeds, that can change fats into fatty acids, glycerin, and sugar.

**Lipid Metabolism** - the process of turning any one of a group of organic compounds including fats, oils, waxes, and sterols into energy and living tissue. These compounds are characterized by an oily feeling, solubility in fat solvents such as chloroform, benzene, or ether, and insoluble in water.

**Lipolysis** - the breakdown or dissolution of fat, as by the action of lipase.

**Listless** - seeming too tired to care about anything; not interested in things; not caring to be active.

**Lumen - 1.** the space within a tubular organ, such as a blood vessel. **2.** a unit of light, equivalent to the amount of light given out per second, through an angle by a point source of one candela radiating in all directions. **3.** the central cavity or space within the wall of a cell.

**Malignant** - very dangerous; causing or threatening to cause death. Also see tumor.

**Mania** - a kind of insanity characterized by great excitement; form or phase of mental disorder, characterized by extremes of joy or rage, uncontrolled and often violent activity, extravagant and irregular speech, and the like, often followed by depression. It is a recurring state in manic - depressive psychosis.

**Masculinizing** - to produce masculine characteristics in (a female).

**Menses** - the discharge of bloody fluid from the uterus that normally occurs approximately every four weeks between puberty and meno-pause.

**Menstruation** - the shedding and discharge of a bloody fluid from the uterus; the act or period of menstruating.

**Metabolic** - having to do with or produced by metabolism.

**Metabolism** - the process by which all living things turn food into energy and living tissue. The metabolism food is broken down to produce energy, which is then used by the body to build up new cells and tissues, provide heat, and engage in physical activity. Growth and action depend on metabolism.

**Metabolites** - substances produced by metabolism.

**Morbid** - abnormal.

**Mucous** - containing or secreting mucus.

**Mucous Membrane** - the lining of the nose, throat, anus, and other cavities of the body that are open to the air; tissue containing glands that secrete mucus; mucosa.

**Mucosa** - mucous membrane.

**Mucus** - a slimy substance that is secreted by and moistens and protects the mucous membranes of the body. A cold in the head causes a discharge of mucus.

**Mutism** - inability to speak.

**Narcolepsy** - a disorder characterized by uncontrollable spells of sleepiness in the daytime, occasional loss of muscular power, and paralysis and hallucinations occurring during sleep.

**Nausea** - the feeling that one is about to vomit.

**Nervous System** - a system in animals that coordinates, controls, and regulates various organic activities by means of the reception and transmission of stimuli.

**Neurohormone** - a hormone that stimulates nerve cells or the ncrv-ous system.

**Neuron** - nerve cell; the fundamental cellular unit of the nervous system, consisting of a nucleus with all its processes and extensions; the single unit which, in bundles or large numbers, makes up a nerve and the nervous system.

**Neuronal** - relating to a neuron.

# "Drugs and Beyond"

**Nightshade Family** - a group of dicotyledonous herbs, shrubs, or small trees, many of which contain narcotic or poisonous alkaloids. The family includes potato, tobacco, belladonna, jimson weed, mandrake, tomato, bittersweet, and petunia.

**Norepinephrine** - a synaptic transmitter in both the central and peripheral nervous systems.

**Nystagmus** - the eyeballs rhythmically moving back and forth, either smooth or jerky.

**Obese** - extremely fat.

**Opisthotonos** - a continuous severe spasm of the muscles causing the back to arch back, the head to bend on the neck, the heels to bend back on the legs and the arms and hands to flex rigidly at the joints.

**Oral** - giving a tablet, capsule, solution, or other form of a liquid or solid drug by mouth.

**Organics** - relating to those compounds in which the atoms are linked by covalent bonds, chiefly the compounds of carbon; originally, relating to compounds of natural origin.

**Overactive** - too active; active to excess.

**Overdose** - too big a dose; more than is needed or wanted.

**Palpitations** - perceptible forcible pulsation of the heart, usually with an increase in frequency or force, with or without irregularity in rhythm.

**Paralysis - 1.** a lessening or loss of the power of emotion or sensa-tion in any part of the body. **2.** a condition of helpless lack of activity; state of being helpless; crippling.

**Paranoia** - a form of psychosis in which a person imagines that he is being persecuted or that he is very great or important. People suffering from paranoia maintain their intelligence, although paranoia is a chronic disorder whose symptoms approach schizophrenia the closer the consciousness comes to realizing the conflicts of personality.

**Paraphernalia** - equipment used to take drugs.

**Paresthesia** - an abnormal sensation, such as of burning, pricking, tickling, or tingling.

**Parkinson' s Disease** - a chronic nervous disease, usually occurring late in life, characterized by muscular tremors and weakness, a tendency to walk peculiarly, and a fixity in facial expression.

**Pathogenic** - that which causes disease.

**Pathologic** - due to disease or accompanying disease.

**Penis** - the male organ of copulation. Urine leaves the body of the male mammal through the penis.

**Peptide** - any combination of two or more amino acids in which the carboxyl group of one acid is joined with the amino group of another.

**Peripheral Nervous System** - the nerves of the outer system; not central.

**Pharmaceutical** - pertaining to, using or relating to the art or business of compounding and identifying drugs, and of compounding and dispensing medicines.

**Pharmacology** - the science of drugs, their properties, preparation, uses, and effects.

**Pharmacy** - the art or business of compounding and identifying drugs, and of compounding and dispensing medicines.

**Phlebitis** - inflammation of a vein.

**Photosensitivity** - eyes being more than normally sensitive to light.

**Pituitary** - **1.** having to do with the pituitary gland. **2.** Designating a type of physique, obese and with large bone structure, thought to be caused by excessive secretion of the pituitary gland.

**Pleurisy** - inflammation of the thin membrane covering the lungs and lining the thorax, often marked by fever, chest pains, and difficulty in breathing.

**Pneumonia** - a disease in which the lung or lungs are inflamed. Pneumonia is caused by a bacterium or virus. It is often an acute infection of the lung accompanied by high fever, pain, and severe cough. Pneumonia in both lungs is called double pneumonia.

**Poultice** - a soft, moist mass, especially of mustard, herbs, or flaxseed, applied hot to the body as a medicine.

**Prednisolone** - a powerful steroid hormone, used in treating arthritis, inflammatory diseases, asthma, and certain allergies; metacortandralone.

**Prednisone** - a drug similar to prednisolone, usually administered orally; metacortandracin.

**Priapism** - intentional indecency.

**Prostration** - severely worn out; lack of energy.

**Psychoanalysis** - the examination of a person's mind to discover the unconscious desires, fears, anxieties, or motivating forces which produce certain mental and emotional disorders.

**Psychomotor** - of or having to do with muscular activity directly related to or coming from mental processes.

**Psychoses** - more than one psychosis.

**Psychosis** - any severe form of mental disturbance or disease which may also be associated with physical disease, and which produces deep and far - reaching disruption of normal behavior and normal function.

**Psychotherapy** - a treatment of mental or emotional disorders by psychological means, especially those involving intercommunication, as by psychoanalysis.

**Psychotic** - having a psychosis; insane.

**Pulmonary** - of or having to do with the lungs.

**Putrefaction** - the action or process of decay; rotting.

**Quiescence** - absence of activity; quiet state; stillness; motionless.

**Reagent** - a substance used to detect the presence of other substances by the chemical reactions it causes.

**Resin - 1.** a sticky yellow or brown substance that flows from certain plants and trees, especially the pine and fir. Resin is transparent or translucent, does not conduct electricity, and is used in medicine, varnish, plastics, inks, and adhesives. When pine resin is heated it yields turpentine; the hard yellow substance that remains is called rosin. Copal, rosin, and amber are types of resin. **2.** any one of a large group of resinous substances that are made artificially and are used especially in making plastics.

**Retention** - the keeping in the body of what normally belongs there, especially the retaining of food and drink in the stomach, or of what normally should be discharged, as urine or feces.

**Rheumatism** - a disease with inflammation, swelling, and stiffness of the joints.

**Rhinitis** - inflammation of the mucous membranes of the nose, with a nasal discharge.

**Rigidity** - stiffness, hardness, or tension.

**Schizophrenia** - a form of psychosis in which the patient dissociates himself from his environment and deteriorates in character and personality.

**Sciatica** - pain in a sciatic nerve and its branches, felt on the hip, thigh, and leg.

**Secrete** - to produce and discharge.

**Secretion** - *1.* a substance that is secreted by some part of an animal or plant. *2.* the act or process of producing and secreting such a substance.

**Sedative** - a medicine that lessens nervousness, pain, or excitement.

**Sedative-Hypnotic** - a drug that temporarily slows down the central nervous system, used mostly to bring sleep and calm nervousness.

**Seizure** - an attack; the sudden onset of a disease or of certain symptoms, such as convulsions.

**Sepsis** - presence of various pus-forming and other pathogenic organisms, or other toxins, in the blood or tissues.

**Septic** - causing infection or putrefaction.

**Septic Shock** - associated with sepsis, usually associated with abdominal and pelvic infection complicating trauma or operations.

**Serotonin** - a substance in the blood that causes blood vessels to constrict and aids in blood clotting.

**Shock** - a condition of physical collapse or depression, together with a sudden drop in blood pressure, often resulting in unconsciousness. Shock may set in after a severe injury, a great loss of blood, or a sudden emotional disturbance.

# "Drugs and Beyond"

**Snort - 1.** to force the breath violently through the nose with a loud, harsh sound. **2.** to snuff or inhale a narcotic or any other drug, especially through the nose, which will create a "high" by doing so. *To snort cocaine.*

**Soluble** - that which can be dissolved or made into liquid. *Salt is soluble in water.*

**Spasm** - any involuntary convulsive muscular contraction.

**Sperm** - the fluid of a male that fertilizes the eggs of the female; semen.

**Stabilize** - to prevent changes in, especially further changes.

**Stereotypy** - repetitive behaviors; repeated talking or body movements.

**Sterile** - free from living germs or microorganisms.

**Stimulant** - a food, drug, or medicine that temporarily increases the activity of the body or some part of the body.

**Stupor** - a dazed condition; loss or the lessening of the power to feel.

**Sublingual** - beneath the tongue.

**Succumbed** - to give way; yield; to give in.

**Suppository** - an easily melted cone or cylinder of material mixed with a drug for placing in the rectum, urethra or vagina. Drugs given this way are absorbed into the system.

**Suppressant** - that suppresses (stops) an attack, symptom, reaction, or the like.

**Synapse** - the junction point of two neurons, across which a nerve impulse passes.

**Synaptic** - relating to synapse or synapsis.

**Synthetic** - relating to a substance that is artificial and not natural.

**Systolic Blood Pressure** - pressure caused by the normal, rhythmical contraction of the heart, especially that of the ventricles, when blood is pumped from the heart into the arteries. Systole alternates with diastole, the two together constituting the cardiac cycle.

**Tachycardia** - excessively fast heartbeat.

**Testicle** - either one of the two reproductive glands of a male animal that secrete sperm; testis.

**Testosterone** - a hormone secreted by the testicles or produced synthetically. Testosterone is responsible for the secondary sex characteristics of males. Chemically, it is a white, crystalline steroid.

**Tinnitus** - persistent ringing of the ears.

**Topic** - something which is applied to the body and absorbed through the skin as a medicine. *A poultice is topic.*

**Toxic** - of, having to do with, or caused by a toxin or poison.

**Toxicity** - toxic or poisonous quality; poisonousness.

**Toxin** - any poison formed by an animal or plant organism as a product of its metabolism, especially one of those produced by bacteria.

**Tracheobronchitis** - inflammation of the windpipe and bronchi.

**Tranquilizer** - any one of various drugs for reducing physical or nervous tension, lowering blood pressure, or bringing into balance certain other conditions of the body; ataractic.

**Tremor** - an involuntary shaking or trembling.

**Trip** - effects caused by an hallucinogen.

**Tumor** - an abnormal growth in or on some part that may be benign or malignant. Tumors exhibit laws of growth independent of the surrounding tissue and are characterized by gradual development. Some tumors are thought to be caused by viruses.

**Ulcer** - an open sore on the skin, or within the body, on a mucous membrane. It sometimes discharges pus.

**Urethra** - the duct in most mammals through which urine is discharged from the bladder, and, in males, through which the semen is also discharged.

**Urticaria** - a disease of the skin, characterized by transient eruptions and attend with itching.

**Vasoactive** - acting on the blood vessels, especially by constricting or dilating them.

**Vasoactive Substances** - substances which act on the blood vessels, especially by constricting or dilating them.

# *"Drugs and Beyond"*

**Vasoconstriction** - constriction of the blood vessels, especially by the action of a nerve or drug.

**Vasodilation** - dilation of the blood vessels, especially by a nerve or drug.

**Ventricle** - either of the two lower chambers of the heart that receive blood from the auricles and force it into the arteries.

**Visine** (*Oxymetazoline*) - is a liquid used to relieve redness due to minor eye irritations, such as those caused by colds, dust, wind, smog, pollen, swimming, or wearing contact lenses. When certain drugs are used (i.e. - marijuana) they can cause redness of the eyes. Users sometimes use visine to avoid detection of the use of such drugs.

**Vulva** - the external genital organs of the female.

**Withdrawal** - the act of depriving or state of being deprived of the use of narcotic drugs. A condition of physical distress in an addict suddenly deprived of narcotic drugs.

# Drug Addiction Rehabilitation and Information <u>Centres</u>

**Division of Alcoholism and Drug Abuse**
**Department of Mental Health**
135 S. Union St.
Montgomery, Alabama 36130
(205) 265-2301

**Department of Health and Social Services**
**Office of Alcoholism and Drug Abuse**
Pouch H-05-F
Juneau, Alaska 99811
(907) 586-6201

**Alberta Alcohol and Drug Abuse Commision (AADAC)**
10909 Jasper Avenue
Edmonton, Alberta
T5J 3M9
(403) 427-0116

**Mental Health Clinic**
Government of America Samoa
Pago Pago, American Samoa 96799

**3HO Super Health**
1050 North Cherry Avenue
Tucson, Arizona 85719

**Drug Abuse Section**
**Department of Health Sciences**
2500 E. Van Buren
Phoenix, Arizona 85008
(602) 255-1239

# "Drugs and Beyond"

## Office on Alcohol and Drug Abuse Prevention
1515 W. 7th Ave.
Little Rock, Arkansas 72205
(501) 371-2604

## Alcohol and Drug Programs of B.C.
Ministry of Health
6th Floor, 1019 Wharf Street
Victoria, British Columbia
V8V 1X4
(604) 387-4738

## Betty Ford Center
39000 BobHope Drive
Rancho Mirage, California 92270
1-800-392-7540 (California Residents Only)
1-800-854-9211 (Out of State)

## Department of Alcohol and Drug Abuse
111 Capital Mall
Sacramento, California 95814
(916) 445-1940

## Haight Ashbury Free Medical Clinic
Educatin Office
409 Clayton Street
San Francisco, California 94117

## Alcoholism and Drug Abuse Prevention
## Department of Health
4210 E. 11th Ave.
Denver, Colorado 80220
(303) 320-8333

## Alcohol and Drug Abuse Council
90 Washington Street
Hartford, Connecticut 06115
(203) 566-4145

## Bureau of Substance Abuse
1901 N. DuPont Hwy.
Newcastle, Delaware 19720

(302) 421-6101

**Mental Health, Alcohol and Addiction Services Branch**
1329 E Street, N.W.
Washington, D.C. 20004
(202) 724-5641

**Coral Ridge Hospital**
Inpatient:
4545 N. Federal Highway
Fort Lauderdale, Florida
(305) 771-2711 Ex. 202
Outpatient:
2000 N.E. 47th Street
Fort Lauderdale, Florida
(305) 771-2711 Ex. 245

**Drug Abuse Program**
1309 Winewood Blvd.
Tallahassee, Florida 32301
(904) 488-0900

**Alcohol and Drug Section**
**Division of Mental Health**
618 Ponce de Leon Ave., N.E.
Atlanta, Georgia 30308
(404) 894-4785

**PRIDE** (**P**arent **R**esources **I**nstitute for **D**rug **E**ducation)
PRIDE is a non-profit organization which provides accurate, up-to-date information about adolescent drug abuse to concerned individuals, parents and young people.
Suite 1216, 100 Edgewood Avenue
Atlanta, Georgia 30303
(404) 658-2548
1-800-241-7946
In Canada: PRIDE Canada Inc. 1-800-667-3747

**Mental Health & Substance Abuse Agency**
P.O. Box 20999
Guam, Guam 96921

# "Drugs and Beyond"

**Alcohol and Drug Abuse Branch**
1270 Queen Emma Street
Honolulu, Hawaii 96813
(808) 548-7655

**Bureau of Substance Abuse**
**Department of Health & Welfare**
700 W. State
Boise, Idaho 83720
(208) 384-7706

**Dangerous Goods Commision**
300 N. State Street
Chicago, Illinois 60610
(312) 822-9860

**National Association for Perinatal Addiction Reasearch**
**and Education**
11 East Hubbard Street, Suite 200
Chicago, Illinois 60611
312-329-2512
1-800-638-BABY - crack/cocaine baby help line

**Division of Addiction Services**
**Department of Mental Health**
5 Indiana Square
Indianapolis, Indiana 46204
(317) 633-4477

**Department of Substance Abuse**
418 Sixth Ave.
Des Moines, Iowa 50319
(515) 281-3641

**Alcoholism & Drug Abuse Section**
2700 W. Sixth Street
Topeka, Kansas 66606
(913) 296-3925

**Alcohol and Drug Branch**
**Bureau of Health Sciences**
275 E. Main Street
Frankfort, Kentucky 40621
(502) 564-7450

**Bureau of Substance Abuse**
**Department of Health and Human Resources**
200 Lafayette Street
Baton Rouge, Louisiana 70801
(504) 342-2575

**Office of Alcoholism and Drug Abuse Prevention,**
**Bureau of Rehabilitation**
32 Winthrop Street
Augusta, Maine 04330

**Alcoholism Foundation of Manitoba (AFM)**
Third Floor, 1031 Portage Avenue
Winnipeg, Manitoba
R3G 0R8
(204) 944-6200

**American Council for Drug Education**
204 Monroe Street, Suite 110
Rockville, Maryland 20850
1-800-488-3748

**State Drug Abuse Administration**
201 W. Preston Street
Baltimore, Maryland 21201
(301) 383-7404

**Division of Drug Rehabilitation**
160 N. Logan Street
Boston, Massachusetts 02114
(617) 727-8614

**Office of Substance Abuse Services**
**Department of Public Health**
3500 N. Logan Street

Lansing, Michigan 48914
(517) 373-8600

**Chemical Dependency Program Division**
**Department of Public Welfare**
658 Cedar
St. Paul, Minnesota 55155
(612) 296-4610

**Division of Alcohol & Drug Abuse**
**Department of Mental Health**
619 Robert E. Lee State Office Building
Jackson, Mississippi
(601) 354-7031

**Division of Alcoholism and Drug Abuse**
**Division of Mental Health**
2002 Missouri Blvd.
Jefferson City, Missouri 65101
(314) 751-4942

**Alcohol & Drug Abuse Division**
**Department of Institutions**
Helena, Montana 59601
(406) 449-2827

**Commission on Drugs**
P.O. Box 94726
Lincoln, Nebraska 68509
(402) 471-2691

**Bureau of Alcohol & Drug Abuse**
505 E. King Street
Carson City, Nevada 89710
(702) 885-4790

**Public Health and Medical Services**
**Department of Health and Community Services**
**Health Promotion and Disease Prevention**
P.O. Box 5100
Fredricton, New Brunswick
E3B 5J8

(506) 453-3092

**Program on Alcohol & Drug Abuse**
61 S. Spring Street
Concord, New Hampshire 03301
(603) 271-3531

**Division of Narcotic & Drug Abuse Control**
129 E. Hanover Street
Trenton, New Jersey 08625
(609) 292-5760

**Substance Abuse Bureau
Behavioral Services Division**
P.O. Box 968
Santa Fe, New Mexico 87503
(505) 827-5271

**Comprehensive Medical Care**
76 Louden Avenue
Amityville, New York
(516) 789-7031

**Division of Substance Abuse Services**
Executive Park S., Box 8200
Albany, New York 12203
(518) 457-7629

**Drug Dependency Services**
P.O. Box 8700
St. John's, Newfoundland
A1B 4J6
(709) 729-0623

**Alcohol and Drug Abuse Section
Department of Human Resources**
325 N. Salisbury Street
Raleigh, North Carolina 27611
(919) 733-6650

# "Drugs and Beyond"

**Division of Alcohol & Drug Abuse**
909 Basin Ave.
Bismarck, North Dakota 58505
(701) 224-2767

**Alcohol, Drugs and Community Mental Health Services of NWT**
P.O. Box 1320
6th Floor, Precambrian Building
Yellowknife, Northwest Territories
X1A 2L9
(403) 920-6255

**Nova Scotia Department of Health Drug Dependency Services**
Suite 314, Lord Nelson Building
5675 Spring Garden Road
Halifax, Nova Scotia
B3J 1H1
(902) 424-4270

**Bureau of Drug Abuse**
65 S. Front Street
Columbus, Ohio 43215
(614) 466-9023

**Drug Abuse Services**
**Department of Mental Health**
P.O. Box 53277, Capitol Station
Oklahoma City, Oklahoma 73152
(405) 521-2811

**Addiction Research Foundation of Ontario (ARF)**
33 Russell Street
Toronto, Ontario
M5S 2S1
(416) 595-6000

**Drug Abuse Program**
**Mental Health Division**
2575 Bittern Street, N.E.
Salem, Oregon 97310
(503) 378-2163

**Natural College of Naturopathic Medicine**
11231 Southeast Market Street
Portland, Oregon 07216

**Governor's Council on Drug & Alcohol Abuse**
2102 N. Front Street
Harrisburg, Pennsylvania 17120
(717) 787-9857

**Addiction Services of PEI**
**Department of Health and Social Services**
P.O. Box 37
65 McGill Avenue
Charlottetown, Prince Edward Island
C1A 7K2
(902) 368-4120

**Department of Addiction Control Services**
Box B-Y, Rio Piedras Station
Rio Piedras, Puerto Rico 00928
(809) 763-5014

**Ministere de la Sante' et des Services Sociaux**
Government du Quebec
1005 chemin Ste-Foy
Qucbec, Quebec
G1S 4N4
(418) 643-9887

**Division of Substance Abuse**
**Rhode Island Medical Center**
303 General Hospital
Cranston, Rhode Island 02920
(401) 464-2091

## *"Drugs and Beyond"*

**Saskatchewan Alcohol and Drug Abuse Commission (SADAC)**
1942 Hamilton Street
Regina, Saskatchewan
S4P 3V7

**Commission on Alcohol & Drug Abuse**
3700 Forest Drive
Columbia, South Carolina 29204
(803) 758-2521

**Division of Drugs & Substance Control**
Joe Foss Building
Pierre, South Dakota 57501
(605) 773-3123

**Alcohol & Drug Abuse Services**
501 Union Building
Nashville, Tennessee 37219
(615) 741-1921

**Drug Abuse Prevention Division**
**Department of Community Affairs**
P.O. Box 13166
Austin, Texas 78711
(512) 475-6351

**Health Services**
**Office of the High Commisioner**
Saipan, Trust Territories 96950
FTS 8-556-0220

**Division of Alcoholism & Drugs**
P.O. Box 2500
Salt Lake City, Utah 84110
(801) 533-6532

**Alcohol & Drug Abuse Division**
**Department of Social & Rehabilitation Services**
State Office Building
Montpeller, Vermont 05602
(802) 241-2170

**Division of Mental Health, Alcoholism and Drug Dependency**
P.O. Box 520, Christiansted
St. Croix, Virgin Islands 00820
(809) 774-4888

**Division of Substance Abuse**
**State Department of Mental Health**
P.O. Box 1797
Richmond, Virginia 23214
(804) 786-5313

**Alternatives In Medicine**
1200 Tower Building
7th Avenue and Olive Way
Seattle, Washington 98101
(206) 467-1818

**Bureau of Alcoholism & Substance Abuse**
**Department of Social and Health Services**
Department of Social and Health Services Office Building
Olympia, Washington 98504
(206) 753-3073

**John Bartyr College**
144 N.E. 54th Street
Seattle, Washington 98105

**Division of Alcohol and Drug Abuse**
**State Capitol**
1800 Kanawha Blvd. E.
Charleston, West Virginia 25305
(304) 348-3616

**Bureau of Alcohol and Other Drug Abuse**
One W. Wilson Street
Madison, Wisconsin 53702
(608) 266-2717

# "Drugs and Beyond"

**Substance Abuse Programs**
Hathaway Building
Cheyenne, Wyoming 82002
(307) 777-7118

**Alcohol and Drug Services**
**Yukon Department of Health and Human Resources**
P.O. Box 2703
6118 - 6th Avenue
Whitehorse, Yukon
Y1A 1H5
(403) 667-5777

**National Council on Alcoholism and Drug Dependents**
1-800-NCA-CALL or 1-800-622-2255

**The United Way of America**
The United Way of America provides many different types of services, including substance abuse and prevention. Check the yellow pages for your area- and look under "U" for local affiliates.

# BIBLIOGRAPHY

Mayer, Jean. - *A Diet for Living.* New York: David McKay, 1975.

Rubinstein, Morton K. - *A Doctor's Guide to Non-Prescription Drugs.* New York: New American Library, 1977.

Billups, Norman F. - *American Drug Index 1982.* Philadelphia: J. B. Lippincott Company, 1982.

Julien, Robert M. - *A Primer of Drug Action - second edition.* San Francisco, U.S.A.: W.H. Freeman and Company, 1975.

Airola, Paavo. - *Are You Confused?* Pheonix, AZ: Health Plus, 1972.

Blau, Sheldon Paul, and Shultz, Dodi. - *Arthritis.* New York: Doubleday, 1973.

Howe, Phyllis S. - *Basic Nutrition in Health and Disease - 6th edition.* Philadelphia: W. B. Saunders Co., 1976.

DiPalma, J. R. - *Basic Pharmacology in Medicine.* New York: McGraw-Hill, 1976.

American National Red Cross. - *Blood: The River of Life.* Washington, DC: 1976.

Abrahamson, E. M., and Pezet, A. W. - *Body, Mind and Sugar.* New York: Avon Books, 1977.

United Nations. Food and Agriculture Organization. - *Calorie Requirements.* 1957, 1972.

Washton, A. M. and Gold, M. S. - *Cocaine: A Clinician's Handbook.* New York: The Guilford Press, 1987.

Redda, K. K., Walker, C. A. and Barnett, G. - *Cocaine, Marijuana, Designer Drugs: Chemistry, Pharmacology and Behavior.* Boca Ration: CRC Press, 1989.

# "Drugs and Beyond"

Stone, Fromme & Kagan. - *Cocaine Seduction And Solution.* NY: Clarkcon, Potter, 1984.

Phillips, Joel L., and Wynne, Ronald D. - *Cocaine: The Mystique and The Reality.* New York: Avon Books, 1980.

Beattie, Melody. - *Codependent No More.* New York: Harper & Row, 1987.

Addiction Research Foundation. - *Coffee, Tea, and Me, And....* Toronto, Canada: Alcoholism and Drug Addiction Research Foundation, 1980.

The United States Pharmacopeial Convention, Inc. and Consumer Reports Books. - *Complete Drug Reference - 1993 edition.* Yonkers, NY: Consumers Union, 1992.

*Consumer Reports 38.* "The U.S. Food and Drug Administration: On Food and Drugs.", March 1973.

"Marijuana: The Health Questions." - *Consumer Reports* 40, March 1975.

Krupp, M.A., and Chatton, M.J. - *Current Medical Diagnosis and Treatment.* Los Altos, CA: Long Medical Publications, 1983.

The Drug Abuse Survey Project. *Dealing with Drug Abuse.* A report to the Ford Foundation. New York: Praeger, 1972.

New York State Society Drug Abuse Committee. - *Desk Reference on Drug Misuse and Abuse.* New York, 1981.

Gomez, Joan and Gerch, Marvin J. - *Dictionary of Symptoms.* New York: Stein and Day, 1963.

Martin, Alice A., and Tenenbaum, Frances. - *Diet Against Disease.* Boston: Houghton Mifflin, 1980.

Rosenberg, Harold, and Feldzaman, A. N. - *Doctor's Book of Vitamin Therapy: Megavitamins for Health.* New York: Putnam, 1974.

CBC Prime Time News. - *Documentary: "White Poison."* Canada: Canadian Broadcasting Corporation, Transcripts for: March 16, 1994.

Atkins, Robert C. - *Dr. Atkins' Diet Revolution.* New York: David McKay, 1972.

Schuckit, M. A. - *Drug and Alcohol Abuse: A Clinical Guide to Diagnosis and Treatment.* New York: Plenum Medical Book Co., 1979.

Simpson, L. L., ed. - *Drug Treatment of Mental Disorders.* New York: Raven Press, 1976.

Seymour, Richard B. and Smith, David E., M.D. - *Drugfree.* New York: Sarah Lazin Books, 1987.

Jones, K. L., Shainberg, L. W., Byer, C. O. - *Drugs and Alcohol.* New York: Harper & Row, 1969.

Irwin, Samuel, Ph.D. - *Drugs of Abuse: An Introduction to Their Actions & Potential Hazards.* U.S.A.: The Student Association for the Study of Hallucinogens, 1970.

MartinMindell, Earl. - *Earl Mindell' s New and Revised Vitamin Bible.* New York, U.S.A.: Warner Books Inc., 1979.

Mindell, Earl. - *Earl Mindell' s Pill Bible.* New York, U.S.A.: Paperjacks Ltd., 1988.

Manahan, William, M.D. - *Eat For Health.* CA: H.J. Kramer, 1988.

Fredericks, Carlton. - *Eating Right For You.* New York: Grosset and Dunlap, 1972.

Ketcham, Katherine and Mueller, L. Anne, M.D. - *Eating Right To Live Sober.* New York: Writers House, 1983.

Peroutka, Stephen, J. - *Ecstacy: The Clinical, Pharmacological and Neurotoxicological Effects Of The Drug MDMA.* Boston/Dordrecht, London: Kluwer Academic Publishers, 1990.

Bevan, J. A. - *Essentials of Pharmacology - 2nd edition.* New York: Harper & Row, 1976.

# "Drugs and Beyond"

Burns, David D. - **Feeling Good, The New Mood Therapy.** New York: New American Library, 1980.

LaDu, B. N., Mandel, H. G. and Way, E. L. - **Fundamentals of Drug Metabolism and Drug Disposition.** Baltimore: Williams and Wilkins, 1971.

Pearson, Durk and Shaw, Sandy. - **Good News for Smokers.** Huntington Beach, CA: The International Institute of Natural Health Sciences, Inc., 1980.

Martin, Marvin. - **Great Vitamin Mystery.** Rosemont, IL: National Dairy Council, 1978.

Roe, Daphne A. - **Handbook: Interactions of Selected Drugs and Nutrients in Patients.** Chicago: The American Dietic Association, 1982.

Quillin, Patrick, Ph.D., R.D. - **Healing Nutrients.** New York: Vintage, 1989.

Weil, Andrew. - **Health and Healing: Understanding Conventional and Alternative Medicine.** Boston: Houghton Mifflin, 1983.

Kordel, L. - **Health Through Nutrition.** New York: MacFadden-Bartell, 1971.

Burton, Benjamin. - **Human Nutrition - 3rd edition.** New York: McGraw - Hill, 1976.

Airola, Paavo. - **Hypoglycemia, A Better Approach.** Pheonix, AZ: Health Plus, 1977.

Nutrition Foundation. - **Index of Nutrition Education Materials.** Washington, DC: 1977.

Smith, D. E. and Gay, G. R. - **It's So Good, Don't Even Try It Once: Heroin in Perspective.** Englewood Cliffs, N.J.: Prentice-Hall, 1972.

Brody, Jane. - **Jane Brody's Good Food Book: Living The High Carbohydrate Way.** New York: Norton, 1985.

Flynn, Magaret A. "The Cholesterol Contraversy." - *Journal of the American Pharmacy.* NS18 (May 1978).

Clark, Linda. - *Know Your Nutrition.* New Canaan, CT: Keats Publishing Co., 1973.

Brecher, E. M. - *Licit & Illicit Drugs. The Consumers Union Report on Narcotics, Stimulants, Depressants, Inhalants, Hallucinogens, and Marijuana - Including Caffeine, Nicotine, and Alcohol.* Boston: Little, Brown, 1972.

Ludwig, A. M., Levine, J. and Stark, L. H. - *LSD and Alcoholism: A Clinical Study of Treatment Efficacy.* Springfield, Ill.: C. C. Thomas, 1970.

The Reader's Digest Association - *Magic and Medicine of Plants.* U.S.A., 1986.

Nahas, G. G. - *Marihuana: Deceptive Weed.* New York: Raven Press, 1974.

Mikuriya, T. H., ed. - *Marijuana: Medical Papers, 1839-1972.* Oakland, CA.: Medi-Comp Press, 1973.

Mayo Foundation for Medical Education and Research. - *Mayo Clinic Family Health Book.* New York: William Morrow and Company, 1990.

Goth, A. - *Medical Pharmacology - 7th edition.* St. Louis: C. V. Mosby, 1975.

Adams, Ruth, and Murray, Frank. - *Minerals: Kill or Cure.* New York: Larchmont Books, 1976.

Goodhart, Robert S. and Shills, Maurice E. - *Modern Nutrition in Health and Disease - 5th edition.* Philadelphia: Lea and Febiger, 1973.

Lennard & Epstein. - *Mystification And Drug Misuse.* CA: Jossey-Bass Inc., 1971.

Cituk, Kathy and Finnegan, John. - *Natural Foods and Good Cooking.* CA: Elysian Arts, 1989.

# "Drugs and Beyond"

Lucas, Richard. - *Nature's Medicines.* New York: Prentice-Hall, 1966.

Prevention Magazine. - *New Encyclopedia Of Common Diseases.* Pennsylvania: Rodale, 1984.

Burack, Richard, with Fox, Fred J. - *New Handbook of Prescription Drugs - revised.* New York: Ballantine Books, 1980.

Mann, M. - *New Primer on Alcoholism - 2nd edition.* New York: Holt, Rinehart and Winston, 1968.

Frank, Benjamin S. - *No Aging Diet.* New York: Dial, 1976.

Kirschmann, John D. and Dunne, Lavon J. - *Nutrition Almanac.* New York: McGraw-Hill, 1984.

Pfeiffer, Carl C. Ph.D., M.D. - *Nutrition And Mental Illness.* Vermont: Healing Arts, 1987.

Cooper, Barber, Mitchell, Rynberge and Green. - *Nutrition in Health and Disease.* New York: Lippincott, 1963.

Stimmel, B. - *Pain, Analgesia and Addiction: The Pharmacologic Treatment of Pain.* New York: Raven Press, 1983.

Mason, David, and Dyller, Fran. - *Pharmaceutical Dictionary and Reference for Prescription Drugs.* New York: Playboy Paperbacks, 1981.

Usdin, Earl; Eckert, Helmut; Forest, Irene, S. - *Phenothiazines and Structurally Related Drugs: Basic and Clinical Studies.* New York, U.S.A.: North Holland, 1980.

Medical Economics. - *Physician's Desk Reference - 36th edition.* Oradell, NJ: Medical Economics Company, 1982.

Medical Economics. - *Physician's Desk Reference - 40th edition.* Oradell, NJ: Medical Economics Company, 1986.

Bricklin, Mark. - *Practical Encyclopedia of Natural Healing.* Emmaus, PA: Rodale Press, 1976.

Bell, C. S., and R. Battjes. - *Prevention Research: Deterring Drug Abuse Among Children and Adolescents.* NIDA Research Monograph 63. Rockville, Md.: U.S. Department of Health and Human Services, Public Health Service, Alcohol, Drug Abuse, and Mental Health Administration, 1985.

Goldstein, A., Aronow, L. and Kalman, S. M. - *Principles of Drug Action - 2nd edition.* New York: Harper & Row, 1974.

Grinspoon, L. and Bakalar, J. B. - *Psychedelic Drugs Reconsidered.* New York: Basic Books, 1979.

Hall, Lindsey and Cohn, Leigh. - *Recoveries.* CA: Gurze Books, 1989.

Finnegan, John and Gray Daphne. - *Recovery From Addiction.* CA: Ten Speed, 1989.

Young, Klein, Beyer. - *Recreational Drugs.* New York: Collier Books, 1977.

Young, Klein, Beyer. - *Recreational Drugs.* New York: Berkley, 1982.

Finnegan, John. - *Regeneration Of Health.* CA: Elysian Arts, 1989.

Meyers, F. H., Jawetz, E. and Goldfein, A. - *Review of Medical Pharmacology - 5th edition.* Los Altos, CA: Lange Medical Publications, 1976.

Sabbag, Robert. - *Snow Blind.* New York: Avon, 1976.

Langer, Stephen E., M.D. - *Solved: The Riddle Of Illness.* Connecticut: Keats, 1984.

Myers, Judy, Ph.D. - *Staying Sober.* New York: Pocket Books, 1987.

Passwater, Richard A. - *Super Nutrition.* New York: Dial, 1975.

Thomas, Clayton L., ed. - *Tabers Cyclopedic Medical Dictionary - 13th edition.* Philadelphia: F. A. Davis, 1977.

Beschner, G. M. and Friedman, A. S. - *Teen Drug Use.* Lexington, Mass.: Lexington Books, 1986.

Musto, D. F. - *The American Disease: Origins of Narcotic Control.* New Haven: Yale University Press, 1973.

Nyholt, David. - *The Athletes Bible.* U.S.A.: Global Health Ltd., 1987.

Coulart, Frances. - *The Caffeine Book.* New York: Dodd Mead & Co., 1984.

Byck, R., ed. - *The Cocaine Papers by Sigmund Freud.* New York: Stonehill Press, 1974.

Rodale, J. I. - *The Complete Book of Minerals for Health - 4th edition.* Emmaus, PA: Rodale Books, 1976.

Null, Gary, and Steve. - *The Complete Book of Nutrition.* New York: Dell, 1972.

Adams, Ruth. - *The Complete Home Guide to All Vitamins.* New York: Larchmont Books, 1972.

Nyholt, David. - *The "Complete" Natural Health Encyclopedia.* U.S.A.: Global Health Ltd., 1993.

Jellinek, E. M. - *The Disease Concept of Alcoholism.* New Haven, Conn.: Hillhouse Press, 1960.

Herer, Jack. - *The Emporer Wears No Clothes - 1993/94 edition.* U.S.A.: HEMP/Queen of Clubs Publishing, 1985.

Stimmel, Barry M.D. - *The Facts About Drug Use.* Binghamptom, U.S.A.: The Haworth Medical Press, 1993.

Lust, John. - *The Herb Book.* New York: Bantam Books, 1974.

Bond, C. Y.; Dobbin, E. V.; Gofman, H. F.; Jones, H. C.; and Lyon, L. - *The Low Fat, Low Cholesterol Diet.* New York: Doubleday, 1971.

Berkow, Robert, ed. - *The Merck Manual - 14th edition.* Rahway, NJ: Merck and Co., 1982.

Brooks, J. E. - *The Mighty Leaf: Tobacco Through the Centuries.* London: Alvin Redman Ltd., 1953.

Pomeranz, Virginia E., and Schultz, Dodi. - *The Mothers' and Fathers' Medical Encyclopedia.* New York: New American Library, 1977.

Hunter, B. T. - *The Natural Foods Primer.* New York: Simon & Schuster, 1972.

Seymour, R., Smith, D., Inaba, D., et al. - *The New Drugs: Look Alikes: Drugs of Deception and Designer Drugs.* Center City: Hazelden Press, 1989.

Brace, Edward R. - *The Pediatric Guide to Drugs and Vitamins.* New York: Dell, 1982.

Graedon, Joe. - *The People's Pharmacy.* New York: St. Martin's Press, 1976.

Mount, Guy. - *The Peyote Book: A Study of Native Medicine - 3rd edition.* Cottonwood, CA: Sweetlight Books, 1993.

Von Brucke, F. T., Hornykiewicz, O. and Sigg, E. B. - *The Pharmacology of Psychotherapeutic Drugs.* New York: Springer-Verlag, 1969.

The United States Pharmacopeial Convention. - *The Physicians' and Pharmacists' Guide to Your Medicines.* New York: Ballantine, 1981.

Silverman, Harold M. and Simon, Gilbert I. - *The Pill Book - 2nd edition.* New York: Bantam Books, 1982.

Hatterer, Lawrence, M.D. - *The Pleasure Addicts.* New York: A.S. Barnes & Co., 1980.

Beck, Deva, R.N. and Beck, James, R.N. - *The Pleasure Connection.* CA: Synthesis, 1987.

# *"Drugs and Beyond"*

Chien, I., Gerard, D. L., Lee, R. S. and Rosenfeld, E. - *The Road to H: Narcotics, Delinquency, and Social Policy.* New York: Basic Books, 1964.

Grinspoon, L. and Hedblom, P. - *The Speed Culture: Amphetamine use and Abuse in America.* Cambridge: Harvard University Press, 1975.

Cohen, Sidney, M.D. - *The Substance Abuse Problems.* New York: Haworth Press, 1981.

Hamaker, John D. - *The Survival Of Civilization.* CA: Hamaker-Weaver, 1982.

Dardis, Tom. - *The Thirsty Muse.* New York: Ticknor & Fields, 1989.

Chishti, Hakim G.M., N.D. - *The Traditional Healer.* Vermont: Healing Arts Press, 1988.

Hughes, Richard. - *The Tranquilizing Of America.* New York: Harcourt Brace Janovich, 1979.

Cahn. - *The Treatment of Alcoholics: An Evaluation Study.* New York: Oxford University Press, 1970.

Nyholt, David. - *The Vitamin & Herb Guide.* U.S.A.: Global Health Ltd., 1987.

Samuels, Mike and Bennett, Hal. - *The Well Body Book.* New York: Random House, 1973.

Linde, Shirley. - *The Whole Health Catalog.* New York: Rawson Associates Publishers, 1977.

Conrad, Barnaby. - *Time Is All We Have.* New York: Dell, 1986.

Milam, James, Dr. and Ketcham, Katherine. - *Under The Influence.* New York: Bantam, 1981.

Cammer, Leonard. - *Up From Depression.* New York: Pocket Books, 1969.

Timberlake, Ian: Windsor Star. - *"U.S. addicts may look north"* Edmonton, AB: *The Edmonton Journal,* Friday, April 22, 1994.

Bailey, Hubert. - *Vitamin E: Your Key to a Healthy Heart.* New York: ARC Books, 1964, 1966.

Katz, Marcella. - *Vitamins, Food, and Your Health.* Public Affairs Committee, 1971, 1975.

Borsaak, Henry. - *Vitamins: What They Are and How They Can Benefit You.* New York: Pyramid Books, 1971.

Schaef, Anne Wilson. - *When Society Becomes An Addict.* CA: Harper & Row, 1987.

Karelitz, Samuel. - *When Your Child Is Ill.* New York: Random House, 1969.

Ebon, Martin. - *Which Vitamins Do You Need?* New York: Bantam Books, 1974.

Seaman, Barbara and Gideon. - *Women and the Crisis in Sex Hormones.* New York: Rawson Associates Publishers, 1977.

Plant, M. - *Women, Drinking, and Pregnancy.* London: Tavistock Publications, 1985.

Beasley, Joseph D., M.D. - *Wrong Diagnosis, Wrong Treatment.* New York: Creative Informatics, 1987.

Hay, Louise L. - *You Can Heal Your Life.* CA: Hay House, 1984.

Page, Melvin E., D.D.S. and Abrams, H. Leon, Jr. - *Your Body Is Your Best Doctor!* Connecticut: Keats, 1972.

Evens, Wayne O., and Cole, Jonathan O. - *Your Medicine Chest.* Boston: Little Brown & Co., 1978.

## *"Drugs and Beyond"*

## *Abused & Misused Drugs* ----- *Complete Index*

## "Drugs and Beyond"

### Volatile Inhalants (Deliriants) ..... 113-117

### Other Drugs .............................. 118-128

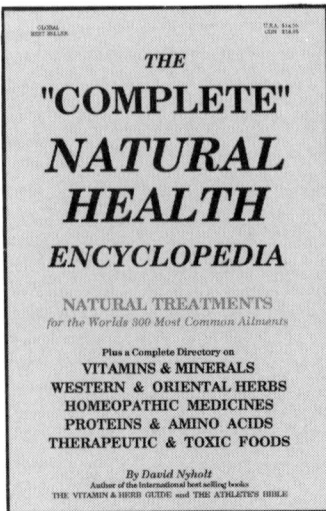

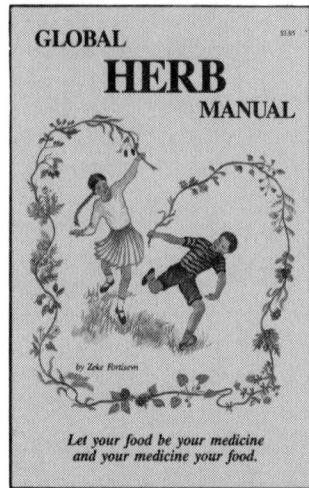

- 222 -

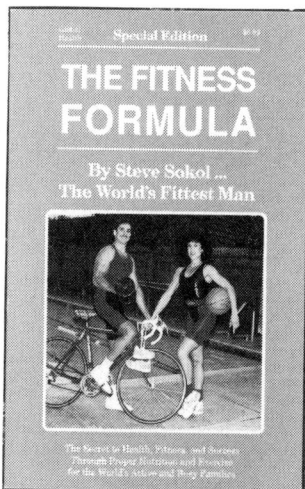

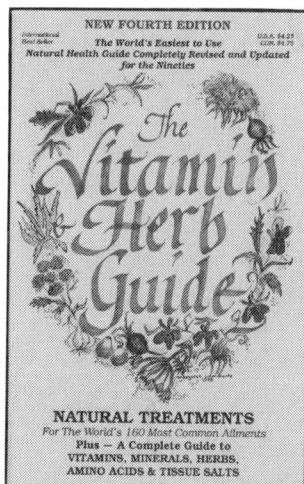

## The Fitness Formula
### A Must For The World's Active and Busy Families
### by Steve Sokol
### $4.95 U.S.A./ $5.95 Cdn.

The Secret to Health, Fitness, and Success. Steve Sokol is not only a talented writer and spokesman for numerous health related associations, but also holds over twenty world fitness records. In this book Steve shares with you his proven techniques designed for people of all skill levels, to increase energy levels, mental alertness, health, and fitness. A sensible plan to feel and look your personal best. Building confidence and success through proper nutrition and exercise.

## The Vitamin & Herb Guide
### Revised Fifth Edition
### By David Nyholt
### $4.95 U.S.A./ $5.95 Cdn.

This highly acclaimed International best seller is the most concise, and easiest to use natural health guide in the world today. Designed to give you more information in less reading time. The quick scan index allows you to find what you want and need to know instantly. features comprehensive quick reference charts on all vitamins, minerals, herbs, amino acids, tissue salts and effective natural treatments for 160 common ailments. That's precisely why busy people around the world rely on - - -
### The Vitamin & Herb Guide.

# *NEW*

*Natural*
*Treatments*
*and*
*Remedies*

BEST GLOBAL SELLER

# THE ATHLETES *BIBLE*

A COMPLETE GUIDE TO

**SUPPLEMENTS**

BUILDER OF CHAMPIONS

AMINOS ---- STEROIDS
STEROLS ---- VITAMIN PAKS
CARBS ---- PROTEINS
HIGH ENERGY & INJURY FIGHTING
SUPPLEMENTS

HOW TO USE – WHAT TO EXPECT

## Natural Treatments & Remedies
**For over 400 of the worlds most common ailments.**
**by Global Health Research**
**$9.95 U.S.A. / $11.95 Cdn.**

This informative and heavily researched book is considered to be the most comprehensive and straight forward natural health guide for the worlds most common ailments on the market today. It has been assembled to give you more information in less reading time and to provide the general public with the latest breakthroughs in natural health science at an affordable price. A must for all families that wish to restore health, prevent premature aging, and prolong life, naturally.

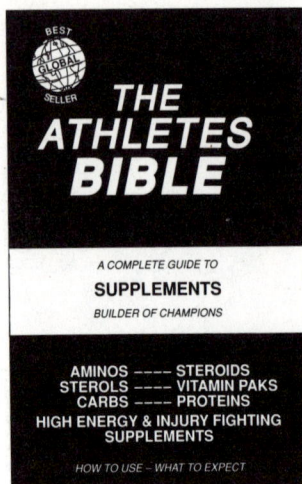

## The Athlete's Bible
**The proper nutrition to boost your athletic abilities.**
**by David Nyholt**
**$9.95 U.S.A./ $11.95 Cdn.**

If you are an Olympic, professional, or recreational athlete, this is the book for you. Concise, up to date information on high performance sport nutrition, aminos, steroids, sterols, vitamins, carbs, proteins, high energy, and injury fighting supplements. Enables you to boost your athletic abilities, promote safe muscle tissue growth, increase strength and stamina. Enhance energy levels through proper nutritional supplementation and reach your highest possible potential, without harmful drugs or chemical additives.